ECG Interpretation

A 2-in-1 Reference for Nurses

ECG Interpretation

A 2-in-1 Reference for Nurses

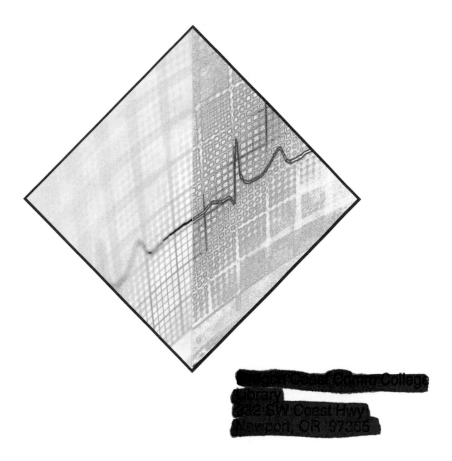

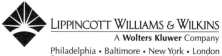

LIPPINCOTT WILLIAMS & WILKINS
A **Wolters Kluwer** Company

Philadelphia • Baltimore • New York • London
Buenos Aires • Hong Kong • Sydney • Tokyo

STAFF

Executive Publisher
Judith A. Schilling McCann, RN, MSN

Editorial Director
H. Nancy Holmes

Clinical Director
Joan M. Robinson, RN, MSN

Senior Art Director
Arlene Putterman

Art Director
Elaine Kasmer

Editorial Project Manager
Jennifer Pierce Kowalak

Clinical Project Managers
Roseanne Hanlon Rafter, RN, MSN, CS;
Mary Perrong, RN, CRNP, MSN, APRN,BC

Editor
Elizabeth Jacqueline Mills

Copy Editors
Kimberly Bilotta (supervisor), Scotti Cohn,
Kelly Taylor, Dorothy P. Terry,
Pamela Wingrod

Designers
PubTech, LLC (project manager)

Digital Composition Services
Diane Paluba (manager), Joyce Rossi Biletz,
Donna S. Morris

Manufacturing
Patricia K. Dorshaw (director), Beth J. Welsh

Editorial Assistants
Megan L. Aldinger, Karen J. Kirk,
Linda K. Ruhf

Indexer
Barbara Hodgson

ECG2IN1 – D N O S A J J M A M F J
07 06 05   10 9 8 7 6 5 4 3 2 1

Library of Congress
Cataloging-in Publication Data

ECG interpretation : a 2-in-1 reference for nurses.
   p. ; cm.
   Includes bibliographical references and index.
   1. Electrocardiography. 2. Nurses. I. Lippincott Williams & Wilkins.
   [DNLM: 1. Electrocardiography — methods — Nurses' Instruction. WG 140 E1717 2006]
RC683.5.E5E253 2008
616.1'207547 — dc22
ISBN 1-58255-395-5 (alk. paper)   2004024449

Contents

Contributors and consultants

Linda S. Baas, RN, PhD, ACNP
Associate Professor and Director, Acute Care Graduate Program
University of Cincinnati College of Nursing

Nancy Bekken, RN, MS, CCRN
Staff Educator, Adult Critical Care
Spectrum Health
Grand Rapids, Mich.

Deirdre Herr Byers, RN, BSN, CCRN
Staff Nurse, CCU
Southeast Georgia Regional Medical Center
Brunswick

Cheryl Westlake Canary, RN, PhD, CS, PN
Assistant Professor
California State University
Fullerton

Louise M. Diehl-Oplinger, RN, MSN, CCRN, APRN,BC
Advanced Practice Nurse
Coventry Cardiology Associates
Phillipsburg, N.J.

Mary Lou Fisher, RN, MSN, CCRN, CRNP
Adult Nurse Practitioner
Johns Hopkins University Hospital
Baltimore

Deborah A. Hanes, RN, MSN, CNS, NP-C
Nurse Practitioner
Cleveland Clinic Foundation

Julene B. Kruithof, MSN, RN, CCRN
Staff Educator, Adult Critical Care – Cardiovascular
Spectrum Health
Grand Rapids, Mich.

Dale Tomlinson Link, RN, MN, CNS
Clinical Care Coordinator, Cardiovascular Services
University of Alabama Hospital
Birmingham

Yun Lu, PharmD, MS, BCPS
Clinical Specialist
Hennepin County Medical Center
Minneapolis

Julia A. McAvoy, RN, MSN, CCRN
RN Specialist
The Washington (Pa.) Hospital

Teresa Palmer, RN, MSN, ANPC, ACNPC
Nurse Practitioner
Rutgers, the State University
New Brunswick, N.J.

Catherine Pence, RN, MSN, CCRN
Assistant Professor
Good Samaritan College of Nursing
Cincinnati

Janis Smith-Love, ARNP-C, MSN, CCRN, CEN
Cardiology Nurse Practitioner
Private Practice of David E. Perloff, MD, FACC, FACP
Fort Lauderdale, Fla.

Mary A. Stahl, RN, MSN, APRN,BC, CCRN
Clinical Nurse Specialist
Saint Luke's Hospital
Kansas City, Mo.

Demetra C. Zalman, RN, BSN, CCRN
Staff Nurse
Hospital of the University of Pennsylvania
Philadelphia

Foreword

In 1902, Willem Einthoven published the first electrocardiogram (ECG). With that publication, the discipline and science of electrocardiology was born. Although amazing advances have been made in the use of ECGs since Einthoven's first publication, the basic notion of recording and displaying the sum of the electrical activity generated by billions of cardiac myocytes remains remarkably similar to that first proposed by him.

Even though the ECG has been in use for more than 100 years, it remains the state-of-the-art instrument for the diagnosis of cardiac arrhythmias, myocardial ischemia and infarction, drug effects, and electrolyte imbalances, and the detection of myocardial structural changes. Further, the ECG is noted for being noninvasive, widely available, easy to use, inexpensive, and reliable.

Unfortunately, many schools offer only an elementary introduction to electrocardiology. As a consequence, most nurses are "self-taught" ECG users who depend on guidance from others and books for their training. Although there are a multitude of ECG books, many of them do little to dispel the confusion faced by most nurses attempting to learn the science and art of ECG interpretation.

ECG Interpretation: A 2-in-1 Reference for Nurses makes the often daunting task of learning to interpret the ECG substantially easier. This text is an exceptional resource for beginners as well as advanced users because of its unique two-column format: an inner one that contains comprehensive text for careful reading and an outer one that summarizes the text to facilitate rapid review. All of the material necessary to become adept at ECG interpretation is contained in this book and includes ECG basics, rhythm strip and 12-lead ECG interpretation, and coverage of arrhythmias and their management.

ECG Interpretation: A 2-in-1 References for Nurses provides an exceptional learning milieu that makes learning ECG interpretation exciting. This book is also distinguished by inclusion of more than 150 rhythm strips that enhance text discussion, treatment algorithms that reflect the latest arrhythmia management guidelines, and helpful tables and illustrations that bring clarity to concepts.

Also included are eye-catching icons that highlight the following information:

◆ *Know-how* — describes specific techniques vital to ECG interpretation.

✦ *Age change*—identifies lifespan differences that may apply to interpreting ECGs.

✦ *Red flag*—highlights warnings for potentially dangerous waveforms.

✦ *Look-alikes*—helps distinguish between two rhythms that appear similar and may easily be confused.

The importance of learning ECG interpretation can't be understated. As the acuity of hospitalized patients increases and hospitals add more monitored beds, the expectation for nurses (in all arenas) to be able to interpret ECGs accurately has risen dramatically. Indeed, as more nurses become nurse practitioners and clinical nurse specialists, they need to learn to interpret ECGs. For all of these reasons this book is a much-needed addition to the literature on ECG interpretation. The contemporary approach used in this text is highly effective and will serve readers well as they strive to become adept in the science and art of electrocardiology.

Willem Einthoven was an amazing visionary, having developed the technology for transmitting his ECGs from the laboratory to the hospital, something that wouldn't become clinical practice for another 50 years. His legacy is well served by nurses who are expert users of the ECG — even though this is surely something even he never envisioned!

Debra K. Moser, RN, DNSc, FAAN
Professor and Linda C. Gill Chair of Nursing
University of Kentucky, College of Nursing
Lexington

ECG Interpretation

A 2-in-1 Reference for Nurses

Cardiac anatomy and physiology

With a good understanding of electrocardiograms (ECGs), you'll be better able to provide expert care to your patients. For example, when you're caring for a patient with an arrhythmia or myocardial infarction, an ECG waveform can help you quickly assess his condition and, if necessary, begin lifesaving interventions.

To build ECG skills, begin with the basics covered in this chapter—an overview of the heart's anatomy and physiology.

CARDIAC ANATOMY

The heart is a hollow, muscular organ that works like a mechanical pump. It delivers oxygenated blood to the body through the arteries. When blood returns through the veins, the heart pumps it to the lungs to be reoxygenated.

LOCATION AND STRUCTURE

The heart lies obliquely in the chest, behind the sternum in the mediastinal cavity, or *mediastinum.* It's located between the lungs and in front of the spine. The top of the heart, called the *base,* lies just below the second rib. The bottom of the heart, called the *apex,* tilts forward and down toward the left side of the body and rests on the diaphragm. (See *Where the heart lies,* page 2.)

The heart varies in size, depending on the person's body size, but is roughly 5″ (12 cm) long and 3½″ (9 cm) wide, or about the size of the per-

Anatomy of the heart
+ Hollow, muscular organ
+ Delivers oxygenated blood to body through arteries
+ When blood returns through veins, pumps it to lungs to be reoxygenated

Location and structure
+ Lies obliquely in chest, behind sternum in mediastinum
+ Varies in size, depending on person's size; usually the size of the person's fist

Where the heart lies

The heart lies within the mediastinum, a cavity that contains the tissues and organs separating the two pleural sacs. In most people, two-thirds of the heart extends to the left of the body's midline.

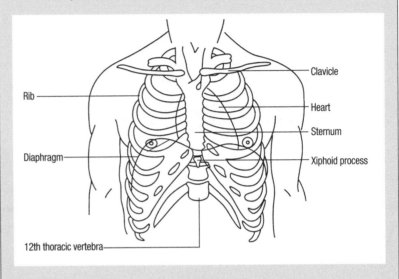

Rib

Diaphragm

12th thoracic vertebra

Clavicle

Heart

Sternum

Xiphoid process

AGE CHANGE

Changes in the heart

THE HEART OF THE OLDER ADULT
As a person ages, his heart usually becomes slightly smaller and loses its contractile strength and efficiency (although exceptions occur in people with hypertension or heart disease). By age 70, cardiac output at rest has diminished by about 30% to 35% in many people.

Irritable with age
As the myocardium of the aging heart becomes more irritable, extra systoles may occur, along with sinus arrhythmias and sinus bradycardias. In addition, increased fibrous tissue infiltrates the sinoatrial node and internodal atrial tracts, which may cause atrial fibrillation and flutter.

THE HEART OF THE CHILD
The heart of an infant is positioned more horizontally in the chest cavity than is an adult's. As a result, the apex is positioned at the fourth left intercostal space. Until age 4, the apical impulse is left of the midclavicular line. By age 7, the heart is located in the same position as an adult's heart is.

Changes in the heart
✦ In older adult, becomes slightly smaller and loses contractile strength and efficiency
✦ In infant, positioned more horizontally in chest cavity

son's fist. The heart's weight, typically 9 to 12 oz (255 to 340 g), varies depending on the person's size, age, sex, and athletic conditioning. An athlete's heart usually weighs more than average, while an elderly person's heart weighs less. (See *Changes in the heart.*)

HEART WALL

The heart wall, encasing the heart, is made up of three layers: epicardium, myocardium, and endocardium. The *epicardium*, the outermost layer, consists of squamous epithelial cells overlying connective tissue. The *myocardium*, the middle and thickest layer, makes up the largest portion of the heart's wall. This layer of muscle tissue contracts with each heartbeat. The *endocardium*, the heart wall's innermost layer, consists of a thin layer of endothelial tissue that lines the heart valves and chambers. (See *Layers of the heart wall.*)

The *pericardium* is a fluid-filled sac that envelops the heart and acts as a tough, protective covering. It consists of the fibrous pericardium and the serous pericardium. The fibrous pericardium is composed of tough, white, fibrous tissue, which fits loosely around the heart and protects it. The serous pericardium, the thin, smooth, inner portion, has two layers:
+ the parietal layer, which lines the inside of the fibrous pericardium

Heart wall

Three layers
+ *Epicardium* — outermost layer
+ *Myocardium* — middle and thickest layer
+ *Endocardium* — innermost layer, consisting of thin layer of endothelial tissue that lines heart valves and chambers

Pericardium
+ Fluid-filled sac that envelops heart and acts as tough, protective coating
+ Consists of fibrous pericardium, (tough, white, fibrous tissue) and serous pericardium (two layers [parietal, visceral])

Layers of the heart wall

This cross section of the heart wall shows its various layers.

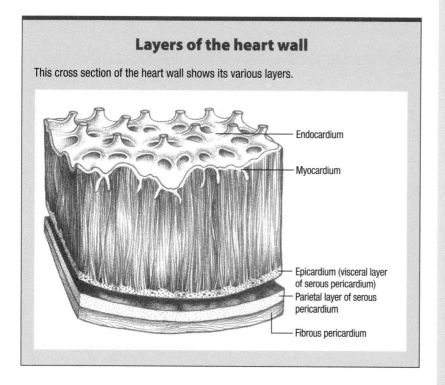

Endocardium

Myocardium

Epicardium (visceral layer of serous pericardium)

Parietal layer of serous pericardium

Fibrous pericardium

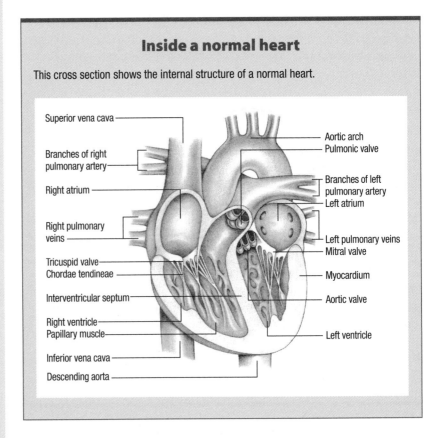

Inside a normal heart

This cross section shows the internal structure of a normal heart.

- Superior vena cava
- Branches of right pulmonary artery
- Right atrium
- Right pulmonary veins
- Tricuspid valve
- Chordae tendineae
- Interventricular septum
- Right ventricle
- Papillary muscle
- Inferior vena cava
- Descending aorta
- Aortic arch
- Pulmonic valve
- Branches of left pulmonary artery
- Left atrium
- Left pulmonary veins
- Mitral valve
- Myocardium
- Aortic valve
- Left ventricle

Heart wall
(continued)

Pericardium
+ Pericardial space separates the visceral and parietal layers and contains 10 to 20 ml of thin, clear, lubricating pericardial fluid

Heart chambers
+ Four chambers: two atria, two ventricles
+ Right atrium receives deoxygenated blood returning from body
+ Left atrium receives oxygenated blood from lungs

+ the visceral layer, which adheres to the surface of the heart.

The pericardial space separates the visceral and parietal layers and contains 10 to 20 ml of thin, clear pericardial fluid that lubricates the two surfaces and cushions the heart. Excess pericardial fluid, a condition called *pericardial effusion,* can compromise the heart's ability to pump blood.

HEART CHAMBERS

The heart contains four chambers—two atria and two ventricles. (See *Inside a normal heart.*) The right atrium lies in front of and to the right of the smaller but thicker-walled left atrium. An interatrial septum separates the two chambers and helps them contract. The right and left atria serve as volume reservoirs for blood being sent into the ventricles. The right atrium receives deoxygenated blood returning from the body through the inferior and superior vena cavae and from the heart through the coronary sinus. The left atrium receives oxygenated blood from the lungs through the four pulmonary veins. Contraction of the atria forces blood into the ventricles.

The right and left ventricles serve as the pumping chambers of the heart. The right ventricle lies behind the sternum and forms the largest part of the heart's sternocostal surface and inferior border. The right ventricle receives deoxygenated blood from the right atrium and pumps it through the pulmonary arteries to the lungs, where it's reoxygenated. The left ventricle forms the heart's apex, most of its left border, and most of its posterior and diaphragmatic surfaces. The left ventricle receives oxygenated blood from the left atrium and pumps it through the aorta into the systemic circulation. The interventricular septum separates the ventricles and helps them pump.

The thickness of a chamber's walls is determined by the amount of pressure needed to eject its blood. Because the atria act as reservoirs for the ventricles and pump the blood a shorter distance, their walls are considerably thinner than the walls of the ventricles. Likewise, the left ventricle has a much thicker wall than the right ventricle because the left ventricle pumps blood against the higher pressures in the aorta. The right ventricle pumps blood against the lower pressures in the pulmonary circulation.

HEART VALVES

The heart contains four valves—two atrioventricular (AV) valves (tricuspid and mitral) and two semilunar valves (aortic and pulmonic). Each valve consists of cusps, or leaflets, that open and close in response to pressure changes within the chambers they connect. The primary function of the valves is to keep blood flowing through the heart in a forward direction. When the valves close, they prevent backflow, or regurgitation, of blood from one chamber to another. Closure of the valves is associated with heart sounds.

The two AV valves are located between the atria and ventricles. The tricuspid valve, named for its three cusps, separates the right atrium from the right ventricle. The mitral valve, sometimes referred to as the *bicuspid valve* because of its two cusps, separates the left atrium from the left ventricle. Closure of the AV valves is associated with S_1, or the first heart sound.

The cusps, or leaflets, of these valves are anchored to the papillary muscles of the ventricles by small tendinous cords called *chordae tendineae*. The papillary muscles and chordae tendineae work together to prevent the cusps from bulging backward into the atria during ventricular contraction. Disruption of either of these structures may prevent complete valve closure, allowing blood to flow backward into the atria. This backward blood flow may cause a heart murmur.

The semilunar valves are so called because their three cusps resemble half moons. The pulmonic valve, located where the pulmonary artery meets the right ventricle, permits blood to flow from the right ventricle to the pulmonary artery and prevents backflow into the right ventricle. The aortic valve, located where the left ventricle meets the aorta, allows blood to flow from the left ventricle to the aorta and prevents blood backflow into the left ventricle.

Heart chambers
(continued)
+ Right ventricle receives deoxygenated blood from right atrium, pumping it to lungs, where it's reoxygenated
+ Left ventricle receives oxygenated blood from left atrium, pumping it into systemic circulation
+ Atria are reservoirs for ventricles (thinner walls than ventricles)
+ Left ventricle has thicker wall than right as it pumps blood against higher pressures in aorta

Heart valves
+ Four valves: two AV valves (tricuspid, mitral), two semilunar valves (pulmonic, aortic)
+ Main function is to keep blood flowing through heart in forward direction

AV valves
+ Tricuspid valve separates right atrium from right ventricle; mitral valve separates left atrium from left ventricle
+ Closure of AV valves associated with S_1

Semilunar valves
+ Pulmonic valve, located where pulmonary artery meets right ventricle
+ Aortic valve, located where left ventricle meets aorta
+ Closure of semilunar valves associated with S_2

Increased pressure within the ventricles during ventricular systole causes the pulmonic and aortic valves to open, allowing ejection of blood into the pulmonary and systemic circulation. Loss of pressure as the ventricular chambers empty causes the valves to close. Closure of the semilunar valves is associated with S_2, or the second heart sound.

BLOOD FLOW THROUGH THE HEART

Understanding the flow of blood through the heart is critical for understanding the overall functions of the heart and how changes in electrical activity affect peripheral blood flow. It's also important to remember that right and left heart events occur simultaneously.

Deoxygenated blood from the body returns to the heart through the inferior vena cava, superior vena cava, and coronary sinus and empties into the right atrium. The increasing volume of blood in the right atrium raises the pressure in that chamber above the pressure in the right ventricle. Then, the tricuspid valve opens, allowing blood to flow into the right ventricle.

The right ventricle pumps blood through the pulmonic valve into the pulmonary arteries and lungs, where oxygen is picked up and excess carbon dioxide is released. From the lungs, the oxygenated blood flows through the pulmonary veins and into the left atrium. This completes a circuit called *pulmonary circulation.*

As the volume of blood in the left atrium increases, the pressure in the left atrium exceeds the pressure in the left ventricle. The mitral valve opens, allowing blood to flow into the left ventricle. The ventricle contracts and ejects the blood through the aortic valve into the aorta. The blood is distributed throughout the body, releasing oxygen to the cells and picking up carbon dioxide. Blood then returns to the right atrium through the veins, completing a circuit called *systemic circulation.*

CORONARY BLOOD SUPPLY

Like the brain and all other organs, the heart needs an adequate supply of oxygenated blood to survive. The main coronary arteries lie on the surface of the heart, with smaller arterial branches penetrating the surface into the cardiac muscle mass. The heart receives its blood supply almost entirely through these arteries. In fact, only a very small percentage of the heart's endocardial surface can obtain sufficient amounts of nutrition directly from the blood in the cardiac chambers. (See *Vessels that supply the heart.*)

Understanding coronary blood flow can help you provide better care to a patient with coronary artery disease because you'll be able to predict which areas of the heart would be affected by a narrowing or occlusion of a particular coronary artery.

Blood flow route through heart
+ Blood returns to heart through inferior vena cava and superior vena cava
+ Right atrium
+ Right ventricle
+ Pulmonary arteries to lungs
+ Pulmonary veins
+ Left atrium
+ Left ventricle
+ Aorta to rest of body

Coronary blood supply
+ Main coronary arteries lie on surface of heart
+ Heart receives its blood supply almost entirely through coronary arteries

Vessels that supply the heart

The coronary circulation involves the arterial system of blood vessels that supply oxygenated blood to the heart and the venous system that removes oxygen-depleted blood from it.

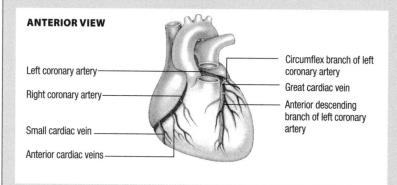

ANTERIOR VIEW

Left coronary artery

Right coronary artery

Small cardiac vein

Anterior cardiac veins

Circumflex branch of left coronary artery

Great cardiac vein

Anterior descending branch of left coronary artery

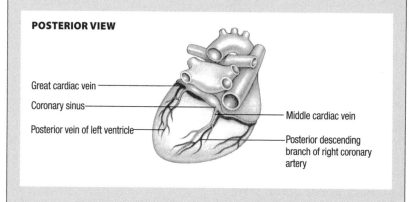

POSTERIOR VIEW

Great cardiac vein

Coronary sinus

Posterior vein of left ventricle

Middle cardiac vein

Posterior descending branch of right coronary artery

Coronary arteries

The left main and right coronary arteries arise from the *coronary ostia*, small orifices located just above the aortic valve cusps. The right coronary artery fills the groove between the atria and ventricles, giving rise to the acute marginal artery and ending as the posterior descending artery. The right coronary artery supplies blood to the right atrium, the right ventricle, and the inferior wall of the left ventricle. This artery also supplies blood to the sinoatrial (SA) node in about 50% of the population and to the AV node in 90% of the population. The posterior descending artery supplies the posterior wall of the left ventricle in 80% to 90% of the population.

Facts about coronary arteries

Right coronary artery

✦ Supplies blood to right atrium, right ventricle, and inferior wall of left ventricle

✦ Posterior descending artery supplies posterior wall of left ventricle

Facts about coronary arteries
(continued)

Left main coronary artery
+ Splits into two major branches: left anterior descending, left circumflex
+ Left anterior descending supplies blood to anterior wall of left ventricle, anterior interventricular septum, bundle of His, right bundle branch, and anterior fasciculus of left bundle branch
+ Left circumflex provides blood to lateral wall of left ventricle and left atrium

The left main coronary artery varies in length from a few millimeters to a few centimeters. It splits into two major branches, the left anterior descending (also known as the *interventricular*) and the left circumflex arteries. The left anterior descending artery runs down the anterior surface of the heart toward the apex. This artery and its branches—the diagonal arteries and the septal perforators—supply blood to the anterior wall of the left ventricle, the anterior interventricular septum, the Bundle of His, the right bundle branch, and the anterior fasciculus of the left bundle branch.

The circumflex artery circles the left ventricle, ending on its posterior surface. The obtuse marginal artery arises from the circumflex artery. The circumflex artery provides oxygenated blood to the lateral wall of the left ventricle, the left atrium, the posterior wall of the left ventricle in 10% of the population, and the posterior fasciculus of the left bundle branch. In about 50% of the population, it supplies the SA node; in about 10% of the population, the AV node.

In most of the population, the right coronary artery is the dominant vessel, meaning the right coronary artery supplies the posterior wall via the posterior descending artery. This is described as *right coronary dominance* or a dominant right coronary artery. Likewise, when the left coronary artery supplies the posterior wall via the posterior descending artery, the terms *left coronary dominance* or dominant left coronary artery are used.

When two or more arteries supply the same region, they usually connect through *anastomoses*, junctions that provide alternative routes of blood flow. This network of smaller arteries, called *collateral circulation*, provides blood to capillaries that directly feed the heart muscle. Collateral circulation often becomes so strong that even if major coronary arteries become narrowed with plaque, collateral circulation can continue to supply blood to the heart.

Coronary artery blood flow

In contrast to the other vascular beds in the body, the heart receives its blood supply primarily during ventricular relaxation or diastole, when the left ventricle is filling with blood. This is because the coronary ostia lie near the aortic valve and become partially occluded when the aortic valve opens during ventricular contraction or systole. However, when the aortic valve closes, the ostia are unobstructed, allowing blood to fill the coronary arteries. Since diastole is the time when the coronary arteries receive their blood supply, anything that shortens diastole, such as periods of increased heart rate or tachycardia, will also decrease coronary blood flow.

In addition, intramuscular vessels are compressed by the left ventricular muscle during systole. During diastole, the cardiac muscle relaxes, and blood flow through the left ventricular capillaries is no longer obstructed.

Facts about coronary artery blood flow
+ Heart receives its blood supply during ventricular relaxation or diastole

Cardiac veins

Just like the other parts of the body, the heart has its own veins, which remove oxygen-depleted blood from the myocardium. Approximately 75% of the total coronary venous blood flow leaves the left ventricle by way of the coronary sinus, an enlarged vessel that returns blood to the right atrium. Most of the venous blood from the right ventricle flows directly into the right atrium through the small anterior cardiac veins, not by way of the coronary sinus. A small amount of coronary blood flows back into the heart through the *thebesian veins*, minute veins which empty directly into all chambers of the heart.

CARDIAC PHYSIOLOGY

In this section, you'll find descriptions of the cardiac cycle; cardiac muscle innervation, depolarization and repolarization; and normal and abnormal impulse conduction.

THE CARDIAC CYCLE

The cardiac cycle includes the cardiac events that occur from the beginning of one heartbeat to the beginning of the next. The cardiac cycle consists of ventricular diastole, or relaxation, and ventricular systole, or contraction. During ventricular diastole, blood flows from the atria through the open tricuspid and mitral valves into the relaxed ventricles. The aortic and pulmonic valves are closed during ventricular diastole. (See *Phases of the cardiac cycle,* page 10.)

During diastole, approximately 75% of the blood flows passively from the atria through the open tricuspid and mitral valves and into the ventricles even before the atria contract. Atrial contraction, or *atrial kick* as it's sometimes called, contributes another 25% to ventricular filling. Loss of effective atrial contraction occurs with some arrhythmias such as atrial fibrillation. This results in a subsequent reduction in cardiac output.

During ventricular systole, the mitral and tricuspid valves are closed as the relaxed atria fill with blood. As ventricular pressure rises, the aortic and pulmonic valves open. The ventricles contract, and blood is ejected into the pulmonic and systemic circulation.

CARDIAC OUTPUT

Cardiac output is the amount of blood the left ventricle pumps into the aorta per minute. Cardiac output is measured by multiplying heart rate times stroke volume. Stroke volume refers to the amount of blood ejected with each ventricular contraction and is usually about 70 ml.

Facts about cardiac veins

+ About 75% of total coronary venous blood flow leaves left ventricle by way of coronary sinus

The cardiac cycle

Ventricular diastole (relaxation)
+ Blood flows from atria into relaxed ventricles
+ About 75% of blood flows passively from atria into ventricles
+ Atrial contraction (atrial kick) contributes another 25% to ventricular filling

Ventricular systole (contraction)
+ Ventricles contract, and blood is ejected into pulmonic and systemic circulation

Cardiac output

+ Measured by multiplying heart rate times stroke volume (amount of blood ejected with each ventricular contraction)

Phases of the cardiac cycle

The cardiac cycle consists of the following phases.

1. Isovolumetric ventricular contraction — In response to ventricular depolarization, tension in the ventricles increases. The rise in pressure within the ventricles leads to closure of the mitral and tricuspid valves. The pulmonic and aortic valves stay closed during the entire phase.

2. Ventricular ejection — When ventricular pressure exceeds aortic and pulmonary artery pressures, the aortic and pulmonic valves open and the ventricles eject blood.

3. Isovolumetric relaxation — When ventricular pressure falls below the pressures in the aorta and pulmonary artery, the aortic and pulmonic valves close. All valves are closed during this phase. Atrial diastole occurs as blood fills the atria.

4. Ventricular filling — Atrial pressure exceeds ventricular pressure, which causes the mitral and tricuspid valves to open. Blood then flows passively into the ventricles. About 70% of ventricular filling takes place during this phase.

5. Atrial systole — Known as the *atrial kick,* atrial systole (coinciding with late ventricular diastole) supplies the ventricles with the remaining 30% of the blood for each heartbeat.

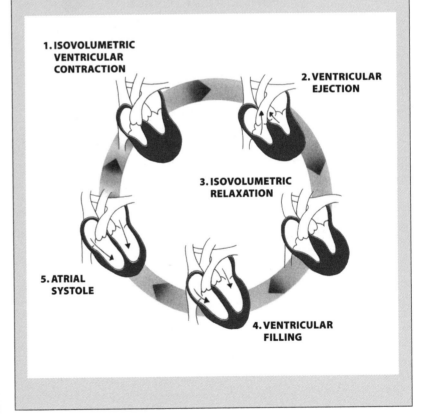

Preload and afterload

Preload refers to a passive stretching exerted by blood on the ventricular muscle fibers at the end of diastole. According to Starling's law, the more the cardiac muscles are stretched in diastole, the more forcefully they contract in systole.

Afterload refers to the pressure that the ventricles need to generate to overcome higher pressure in the aorta to eject blood into the systemic circulation. This systemic vascular resistance corresponds to the systemic systolic pressure.

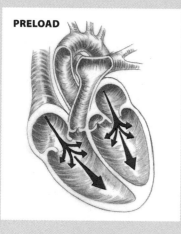

PRELOAD

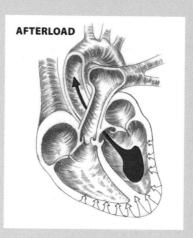

AFTERLOAD

Normal cardiac output is 4 to 8 L per minute, depending on body size. The heart pumps only as much blood as the body requires, based upon metabolic requirements. During exercise, for example, the heart increases cardiac output accordingly.

Three factors determine stroke volume: preload, afterload, and myocardial contractility. (See *Preload and afterload*.) *Preload* is the degree of stretch or tension on the muscle fibers when they begin to contract. It's usually considered to be the end-diastolic pressure when the ventricle has become filled.

Afterload is the load or amount of pressure the left ventricle must work against to eject blood during systole and corresponds to the systolic pressure. The greater this resistance, the greater the heart's workload. Afterload is also called the *systemic vascular resistance.*

Myocardial contractility is the ventricle's ability to contract, which is determined by the degree of muscle fiber stretch at the end of diastole. The more the muscle fibers stretch during ventricular filling, up to an optimal length, the more forceful the contraction.

Cardiac output
(continued)

Three factors determine stroke volume

+ *Preload*—degree of stretch on muscle fibers when they begin to contract
+ *Afterload*—amount of pressure left ventricle must work against to eject blood during systole
+ *Myocardial contractility*—ventricles ability to contract

Autonomic innervation of the heart

✦ Sympathetic nerve stimulation causes release of norepinephrine, which increases heart rate and accelerates AV node conduction
✦ Parasympathetic stimulation causes release of acetylcholine, which slows heart rate and conduction through AV node

Transmission of electrical impulses

Four key cell characteristics
✦ *Automaticity*—cell's ability to spontaneously initiate an electrical impulse
✦ *Excitability*—cell's ability to respond to an electrical impulse
✦ *Conductivity*—cell's ability to transmit an electrical impulse from one cell to another
✦ *Contractility*—cell's ability to contract

Depolarization and repolarization

✦ Cardiac cells at rest are considered polarized
✦ Upon stimulus, ions cross cell membrane, causing an action potential (depolarization)
✦ After depolarization, cell attempts to return to its resting state (repolarization)

AUTONOMIC INNERVATION OF THE HEART

The two branches of the autonomic nervous system—the sympathetic (or *adrenergic*) and the parasympathetic (or *cholinergic*)—abundantly supply the heart. Sympathetic fibers innervate all the areas of the heart, while parasympathetic fibers primarily innervate the sinoatrial (SA) and atrioventricular (AV) nodes.

Sympathetic nerve stimulation causes the release of norepinephrine, which increases the heart rate by increasing SA node discharge, accelerates AV node conduction time, and increases the force of myocardial contraction and cardiac output.

Parasympathetic (vagal) stimulation causes the release of acetylcholine, which produces the opposite effects. The rate of SA node discharge is decreased, thus slowing heart rate and conduction through the AV node, and reducing cardiac output.

TRANSMISSION OF ELECTRICAL IMPULSES

In order for the heart to contract and pump blood to the rest of the body, an electrical stimulus needs to occur first. Generation and transmission of electrical impulses depend on the four key characteristics of cardiac cells: automaticity, excitability, conductivity, and contractility.

Automaticity refers to a cell's ability to spontaneously initiate an electrical impulse. Pacemaker cells usually possess this ability. *Excitability* results from ion shifts across the cell membrane and refers to the cell's ability to respond to an electrical stimulus. *Conductivity* is the ability of a cell to transmit an electrical impulse from one cell to another. *Contractility* refers to the cell's ability to contract after receiving a stimulus by shortening and lengthening its muscle fibers.

It's important to remember that the first three characteristics are electrical properties of the cells, while contractility represents a mechanical response to the electrical activity. Of the four characteristics, automaticity has the greatest effect on the genesis of cardiac rhythms.

DEPOLARIZATION AND REPOLARIZATION

As impulses are transmitted, cardiac cells undergo cycles of depolarization and repolarization. (See *Depolarization-repolarization cycle.*) Cardiac cells at rest are considered polarized, meaning that no electrical activity takes place. Cell membranes separate different concentrations of ions, such as sodium and potassium, and create a more negative charge inside the cell. This is called the *resting potential*. After a stimulus occurs, ions cross the cell membrane and cause an action potential, or cell depolarization. When a cell is ful-

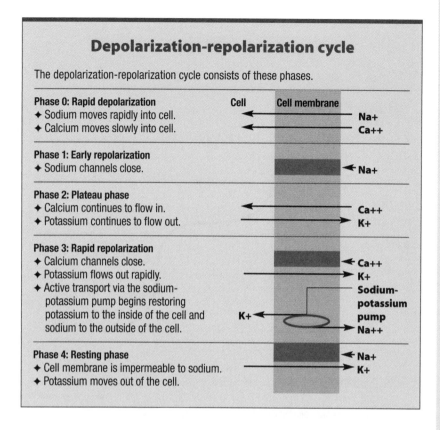

Depolarization-repolarization cycle

The depolarization-repolarization cycle consists of these phases.

Phase 0: Rapid depolarization
- ✦ Sodium moves rapidly into cell.
- ✦ Calcium moves slowly into cell.

Cell | Cell membrane

Na+
Ca++

Phase 1: Early repolarization
- ✦ Sodium channels close.

Na+

Phase 2: Plateau phase
- ✦ Calcium continues to flow in.
- ✦ Potassium continues to flow out.

Ca++
K+

Phase 3: Rapid repolarization
- ✦ Calcium channels close.
- ✦ Potassium flows out rapidly.
- ✦ Active transport via the sodium-potassium pump begins restoring potassium to the inside of the cell and sodium to the outside of the cell.

Ca++
K+
Sodium-potassium pump
K+
Na++

Phase 4: Resting phase
- ✦ Cell membrane is impermeable to sodium.
- ✦ Potassium moves out of the cell.

Na+
K+

---

ly depolarized, it attempts to return to its resting state in a process called *repolarization*. Electrical charges in the cell reverse and return to normal.

A cycle of depolarization-repolarization consists of five phases—0 through 4. The action potential is represented by a curve that shows voltage changes during the five phases. (See *Action potential curves,* page 14.)

During phase 0 (or *rapid depolarization*), the cell receives a stimulus, usually from a neighboring cell. The cell becomes more permeable to sodium, the inside of the cell becomes less negative, the cell is depolarized, and myocardial contraction occurs. In phase 1 (or *early repolarization*), sodium stops flowing into the cell, and the transmembrane potential falls slightly. Phase 2 (the *plateau phase*) is a prolonged period of slow repolarization, when little change occurs in the cell's transmembrane potential.

During phases 1 and 2 and at the beginning of phase 3, the cardiac cell is said to be in its absolute refractory period. During that period, no stimulus, no matter how strong, can excite the cell.

Phase 3 (or *rapid repolarization*) occurs as the cell returns to its original state. During the last half of this phase, when the cell is in its relative refractory period, a very strong stimulus can depolarize it.

Depolarization and repolarization
(continued)

Phases 0 through 4
- ✦ *Phase 0* — cell receives stimulus
- ✦ *Phases 1 and 2* — cell is in absolute refractory period; no stimulus, no matter how strong, can excite cell
- ✦ *Phase 3* — cell is in relative refractory period; however, strong stimulus can depolarize it
- ✦ *Phase 4* — cell is ready for another stimulus
- ✦ Electrical activity of heart represented on ECG

Action potential curves

An action potential curve shows the changes in a cell's electrical charge during the five phases of the depolarization-repolarization cycle. These graphs show electrical changes for nonpacemaker and pacemaker cells.

ACTION POTENTIAL CURVE: NONPACEMAKER CELL

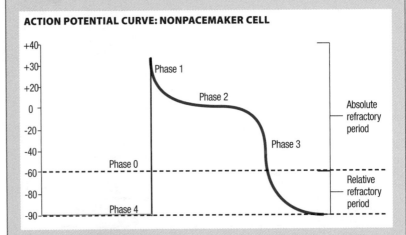

As the graph below shows, the action potential curve for pacemaker cells, such as those in the sinoatrial node, differs from that of other myocardial cells. Pacemaker cells have a resting membrane potential of –60 mV (instead of –90 mV), and they begin to depolarize spontaneously. Called *diastolic depolarization*, this effect results primarily from calcium and sodium leakage into the cell.

ACTION POTENTIAL CURVE: PACEMAKER CELL

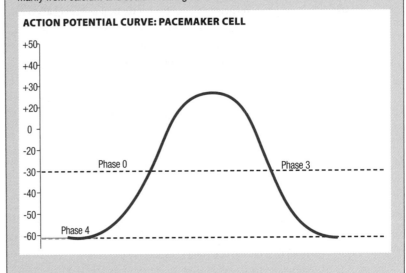

Phase 4 is the resting phase of the action potential. By the end of phase 4, the cell is ready for another stimulus.

The electrical activity of the heart is represented on an ECG. Keep in mind that the ECG represents electrical activity only, not the mechanical activity or actual pumping of the heart.

ELECTRICAL CONDUCTION SYSTEM OF THE HEART

After depolarization and repolarization occur, the resulting electrical impulse travels through the heart along a pathway called the *conduction system*. (See *Cardiac conduction system*, page 16.)

Impulses travel out from the SA node and through the internodal tracts and Bachmann's bundle to the AV node. From there, they travel through the bundle of His, the bundle branches, and finally to the Purkinje fibers.

The SA node, located in the right atrium where the superior vena cava joins the atrial tissue mass, is the heart's main pacemaker. Under resting conditions, the SA node generates impulses 60 to 100 beats/minute. When initiated, the impulses follow a specific path through the heart. Electrical impulses usually don't travel in a backward or retrograde direction because the cells can't respond to a stimulus immediately after depolarization.

From the SA node, an impulse travels through the right and left atria. In the right atrium, the impulse is believed to be transmitted along three internodal tracts. These tracts include the anterior, the middle (or *Wenckebach's*), and the posterior (or *Thorel's*) internodal tracts. The impulse travels through the left atrium via Bachmann's bundle, the interatrial tracts of tissue extending from the SA node to the left atrium. Impulse transmission through the right and left atria occurs so rapidly that the atria contract almost simultaneously.

The AV node is located in the inferior right atrium near the ostium of the coronary sinus. Although the AV node doesn't possess pacemaker cells, the tissue surrounding it, referred to as *junctional tissue,* contains pacemaker cells that can fire at a rate of 40 to 60 beats/minute. As the AV node conducts the atrial impulse to the ventricles, it causes a 0.04-second delay. This delay allows the ventricles to complete their filling phase as the atria contract. It also allows the cardiac muscle to stretch to its fullest for peak cardiac output.

Rapid conduction then resumes through the bundle of His, which divides into the right and left bundle branches and extends down either side of the interventricular septum. The right bundle branch extends down the right side of the interventricular septum and through the right ventricle. The left bundle branch extends down the left side of the interventricular septum and

Electrical conduction system of the heart

+ Impulses travel from SA node (heart's main pacemaker) through internodal tracts and Bachmann's bundle to AV node
+ From AV node, impulses travel through bundle of His, bundle branches, and to Purkinje fibers

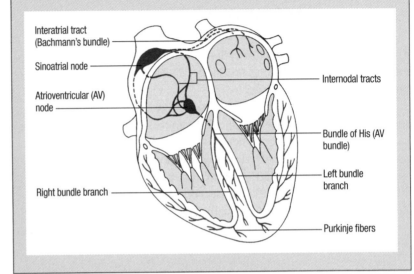

Cardiac conduction system

Specialized fibers propagate electrical impulses throughout the heart's cells, causing the heart to contract. This illustration shows the elements of the cardiac conduction system.

Interatrial tract
(Bachmann's bundle)

Sinoatrial node

Atrioventricular (AV)
node

Right bundle branch

Internodal tracts

Bundle of His (AV
bundle)

Left bundle
branch

Purkinje fibers

Electrical conduction system of the heart
(continued)

✦ SA node generates impulses of 60 to 100 beats/minute
✦ AV node can fire at rate of 40 to 60 beats/minute
✦ Purkinje fibers can fire at rate of 20 to 40 beats/minute

through the left ventricle. As a pacemaker site, the bundle of His has a firing rate between 40 and 60 beats/minute. The bundle of His usually fires when the SA node fails to generate an impulse at a normal rate or when the impulse fails to reach the AV junction.

The left bundle branch then splits into two branches, or fasciculations. The left anterior fasciculus extends through the anterior portion of the left ventricle. The left posterior fasciculus extends through the lateral and posterior portions of the left ventricle. Impulses travel much faster down the left bundle branch, which feeds the larger, thicker-walled left ventricle, than the right bundle branch, which feeds the smaller, thinner-walled right ventricle. The difference in the conduction speed allows both ventricles to contract simultaneously. The entire network of specialized nervous tissue that extends through the ventricles is known as the His-Purkinje system.

Purkinje fibers comprise a diffuse muscle fiber network beneath the endocardium that transmits impulses quicker than any other part of the conduction system. This pacemaker site usually doesn't fire unless the SA and AV nodes fail to generate an impulse or when the normal impulse is blocked in both bundle branches. The automatic firing rate of the Purkinje fibers ranges from 20 to 40 beats/minute.

ABNORMAL IMPULSE CONDUCTION

Causes of abnormal impulse conduction include altered automaticity, retrograde conduction of impulses, reentry abnormalities, and ectopy.

Automaticity, a special characteristic of pacemaker cells, allows them to generate electrical impulses spontaneously. If a cell's automaticity is increased or decreased, an arrhythmia — or abnormality in the cardiac rhythm — can occur. Tachycardia and premature beats are commonly caused by an increase in the automaticity of pacemaker cells below the SA node. Likewise, a decrease in automaticity of cells in the SA node can cause the development of bradycardia or escape rhythms generated by lower pacemaker sites.

Impulses that begin below the AV node can be transmitted backward toward the atria. This backward, or *retrograde*, conduction usually takes longer than normal conduction and can cause the atria and ventricles to lose synchrony.

Reentry occurs when cardiac tissue is activated two or more times by the same impulse. This may happen when conduction speed is slowed or when the refractory periods for neighboring cells occur at different times. Impulses are delayed long enough that cells have time to repolarize. In those cases, the active impulse reenters the same area and produces another impulse.

Injured pacemaker (or nonpacemaker) cells may partially depolarize, rather than fully depolarizing. Partial depolarization can lead to spontaneous or secondary depolarization, repetitive ectopic firings called *triggered activity*.

The resultant depolarization is called *afterdepolarization*. Early afterdepolarization occurs before the cell is fully repolarized and can be caused by hypokalemia, slow pacing rates, or drug toxicity. If it occurs after the cell has been fully repolarized, it's called *delayed afterdepolarization*. These problems can be caused by digoxin toxicity, hypercalcemia, or increased catecholamine release. Atrial or ventricular tachycardias may result.

Abnormal impulse conduction

✦ Causes include altered automaticity, retrograde conduction of impulses, reentry abnormalities, and ectopy

ECG basics

One of the most valuable diagnostic tools available, an electrocardiogram (ECG) records the heart's electrical activity as waveforms. By interpreting these waveforms accurately, you can identify rhythm disturbances, conduction abnormalities, and electrolyte imbalances. An ECG aids in diagnosing and monitoring conditions, such as myocardial infarction and pericarditis.

To interpret an ECG correctly, you must first recognize its key components. Next, you need to analyze them separately. Then you can put your findings together to reach a conclusion about the heart's electrical activity. This chapter explains that analytic process, beginning with some fundamental information about electrocardiography.

The heart's electrical activity produces currents that radiate through the surrounding tissue to the skin. When electrodes are attached to the skin, they sense those electrical currents and transmit them to the electrocardiograph. This electrical activity is transformed into waveforms that represent the heart's depolarization-repolarization cycle.

Myocardial depolarization occurs when a wave of stimulation passes through the heart and causes the heart muscle to contract. Repolarization is the relaxation phase. An ECG shows the precise sequence of electrical events occurring in the cardiac cells throughout that process and identifies rhythm disturbances and conduction abnormalities.

The ECG

+ Records heart's electrical activity as waveforms
+ Identifies rhythm disturbances, conduction abnormalities, and electrolyte imbalances

Leads and planes

- ✦ Electrical currents from heart radiate to skin in many directions
- ✦ Electrodes are placed at different locations to get idea of heart's electrical activity

Leads

- ✦ Provides view of heart's electrical activity between two points
- ✦ Direction of electric current determines how waveforms appear on ECG
- ✦ If current flows along axis toward positive pole of electrode, waveform deflects upward
- ✦ If current flows away from positive pole, waveform deflects downward below baseline
- ✦ If electrical activity is absent or too small to measure, waveform is a straight line

Planes

- ✦ Cross section of heart; provides different view of heart's electrical activity
- ✦ Six limb leads are viewed from frontal plane
- ✦ Six precordial leads are viewed from horizontal plane

LEADS AND PLANES

Because the electrical currents from the heart radiate to the skin in many directions, electrodes are placed at different locations to get a total picture of the heart's electrical activity. The ECG can then record information from different perspectives, which are called *leads* and *planes.*

LEADS

A lead provides a view of the heart's electrical activity between two points, or poles. Each lead consists of one positive and one negative pole. Between the two poles lies an imaginary line representing the lead's axis, a term that refers to the direction of the current moving through the heart. Because each lead measures the heart's electrical potential from different directions, each generates its own characteristic tracing. (See *Current direction and waveform deflection.*)

The direction in which the electric current flows determines how the waveforms appear on the ECG tracing. When the current flows along the axis toward the positive pole of the electrode, the waveform deflects upward and is called a *positive deflection.* When the current flows away from the positive pole, the waveform deflects downward, below the baseline, and is called a *negative deflection.* When the current flows perpendicular to the axis, the wave may go in both directions or be unusually small. When electrical activity is absent or too small to measure, the waveform is a straight line, also called an *isoelectric deflection.*

PLANES

A plane is a cross section of the heart, which provides a different view of the heart's electrical activity. In the frontal plane—a vertical cut through the middle of the heart from top to bottom—electrical activity is viewed from an anterior to posterior approach. The six limb leads are viewed from the frontal plane.

In the horizontal plane—a transverse cut through the middle of the heart dividing it into upper and lower portions—electrical activity can be viewed from a superior or an inferior approach. The six precordial leads are viewed from the horizontal plane.

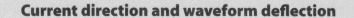

Current direction and waveform deflection

This illustration shows possible directions of electrical current and the corresponding waveform deflections. The direction of the electrical current determines the upward or downward deflection of an electrocardiogram waveform.

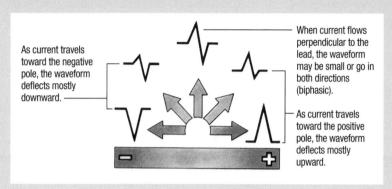

As current travels toward the negative pole, the waveform deflects mostly downward.

When current flows perpendicular to the lead, the waveform may be small or go in both directions (biphasic).

As current travels toward the positive pole, the waveform deflects mostly upward.

TYPES OF ECG RECORDINGS

The two main types of ECG recordings are the 12-lead ECG and the single-lead ECG, commonly known as a *rhythm strip*. Both types give valuable information about the heart's electrical activity.

12-LEAD ECG

A 12-lead ECG records information from 12 different views of the heart and provides a complete picture of electrical activity. These 12 views are obtained by placing electrodes on the patient's limbs and chest. The limb leads and the chest, or precordial, leads reflect information from the different planes of the heart.

Different leads provide different information. The six limb leads—I, II, III, augmented vector right (aV_R), augmented vector left (aV_L), and augmented vector foot (aV_F)—provide information about the heart's frontal plane. Leads I, II, and III require a negative and positive electrode for monitoring, which makes these leads bipolar. The augmented leads—aV_R, aV_L, and aV_F—are unipolar, meaning they need only a positive electrode.

The six precordial or V leads—V_1, V_2, V_3, V_4, V_5, and V_6—provide information about the heart's horizontal plane. Like the augmented leads, the precordial leads are unipolar, requiring only a positive electrode. The nega-

---

Types of ECG recordings

✦ 12-lead ECG and single-lead ECG (rhythm strip)

12-lead ECG

✦ Records information from 12 different views of heart

Six limb leads

✦ Leads I, II, and III — require negative and positive electrode for monitoring, making leads bipolar
✦ aV_R, aV_L, and aV_F — require positive electrode, making these augmented leads unipolar

Six precordial leads

✦ V_1 through V_6 — require positive electrode, making these leads unipolar
✦ Negative pole of these leads, which is in center of heart, is calculated by ECG

tive pole of these leads, which is in the center of the heart, is calculated by the ECG.

SINGLE-LEAD ECG

Single-lead ECG
+ Provides continuous information about heart's electrical activity; used to monitor cardiac status
+ Monitored leads include bipolar leads I, II, and III; other leads include MCL_1 and MCL_6

Single-lead monitoring provides continuous information about the heart's electrical activity and is used to monitor cardiac status. Chest electrodes pick up the heart's electrical activity for display on the monitor. The monitor also displays heart rate and other measurements and prints out strips of cardiac rhythms.

Commonly monitored leads include the bipolar leads I, II, and III. Two other leads, MCL_1 and MCL_6, may also be used. The initials MCL stand for *modified chest lead.* These leads are similar to the unipolar leads V_1 and V_6 of the 12-lead ECG; MCL_1 and MCL_6, however, are bipolar leads.

ECG MONITORING SYSTEMS

ECG monitoring systems

Hardwire monitoring
+ Electrodes are connected directly to cardiac monitor
+ Hardwire monitors are mounted permanently

Telemetry monitoring
+ Small, battery-powered transmitter sends electrical signals to another location, where they're displayed on monitor screen
+ Frees patient from cumbersome wires and cables

The type of ECG monitoring system used — hardwire monitoring or telemetry — depends on the patient's clinical status. With hardwire monitoring, the electrodes are connected directly to the cardiac monitor. Most hardwire monitors are mounted permanently on a shelf or wall near the patient's bed. Some monitors are mounted on an I.V. pole for portability, and some may include a defibrillator.

The monitor provides a continuous cardiac rhythm display and transmits the ECG tracing to a console at the nurses' station. Both the monitor and the console have alarms and can print rhythm strips to show ectopic beats, for example, or other arrhythmias. Hardwire monitors also have the ability to track pulse oximetry, blood pressure, hemodynamic measurements, and other parameters through various attachments to the patient.

Hardwire monitoring is generally used in critical care units and emergency departments because it permits continuous observation of one or more patients from more than one area in the unit. However, this type of monitoring does have disadvantages, including limited mobility because the patient is tethered to a monitor.

With telemetry monitoring, the patient carries a small, battery-powered transmitter that sends electrical signals to another location, where the signals are displayed on a monitor screen. This type of ECG monitoring frees the patient from cumbersome wires and cables and protects him from the electrical leakage and accidental shock occasionally associated with hardwire monitoring.

Telemetry monitoring still requires skin electrodes to be placed on the patient's chest. Each electrode is connected by a thin wire to a small transmitter box carried in a pocket or pouch. Telemetry monitoring is especially useful for detecting arrhythmias that occur at rest or during sleep, exercise, or stressful situations. Most systems, however, can monitor heart rate and rhythm only.

ELECTRODE PLACEMENT

Electrode placement is different for each lead, and different leads provide different views of the heart. A lead may be chosen to highlight a particular part of the ECG complex or the electrical events of a specific area of the heart.

Although leads II, V_1, and V_6 are among the most commonly used leads for continuous monitoring, lead placement is varied according to the patient's clinical status. If your monitoring system has the capability, you may also monitor the patient in more than one lead. (See *Dual lead monitoring*.)

Electrode placement
+ Different for each lead; different leads provide different views of heart
+ With proper capability, allows for monitoring patient in more than one lead

Dual lead monitoring

Monitoring in two leads provides a more complete picture than monitoring in only one lead. With simultaneous dual monitoring, you'll generally review the first lead — usually designated as the primary lead — for arrhythmias.

A two-lead view helps detect ectopic beats or aberrant rhythms. Leads II and V_1 are the leads most commonly monitored simultaneously.

LEAD II

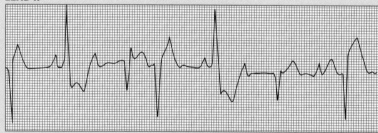

LEAD V_1

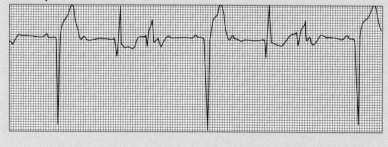

Standard limb leads

Lead I
+ Positive electrode is placed on left arm; negative electrode is placed on right arm
+ Produces positive deflection

Lead II
+ Positive electrode is placed on left leg; negative electrode is placed on right arm
+ Produces positive deflection

Lead III
+ Positive electrode is placed on left leg; negative electrode is placed on left arm
+ Produces positive deflection (usually)

STANDARD LIMB LEADS

All standard limb leads or bipolar limb leads have a third electrode, known as the *ground,* which is placed on the chest to prevent electrical interference from appearing on the ECG recording.

Lead I provides a view of the heart that shows current moving from right to left. Because current flows from negative to positive, the positive electrode for this lead is placed on the left arm or on the left side of the chest; the negative electrode is placed on the right arm. Lead I produces a positive deflection on ECG tracings and is helpful in monitoring atrial rhythms.

Lead II produces a positive deflection. The positive electrode is placed on the patient's left leg and the negative electrode on the right arm. For continuous monitoring, place the electrodes on the torso for convenience, with the positive electrode below the lowest palpable rib at the left midclavicular line and the negative electrode below the right clavicle. The current travels down and to the left in this lead. Lead II tends to produce a positive, high-voltage deflection, resulting in tall P, R, and T waves. This lead is commonly used for routine monitoring and is useful for detecting sinus node and atrial arrhythmias and monitoring the inferior wall of the left ventricle.

Lead III usually produces a positive deflection. The positive electrode is placed on the left leg and the negative electrode on the left arm. Along with lead II, this lead is useful for detecting changes associated with an inferior wall of the left ventricle.

The axes of the three bipolar limb leads — I, II, and III — form a triangle around the heart and provide a frontal plane view of the heart. (See *Einthoven's triangle.*)

Einthoven's triangle

The axes of the three bipolar limb leads (I, II, and III) form a triangle, known as *Einthoven's triangle.* Because the electrodes for these leads are about equidistant from the heart, the triangle is equilateral.

The axis of lead I extends from shoulder to shoulder, with the right arm lead being the negative electrode and the left arm lead being the positive electrode. The axis of lead II runs from the negative right arm lead electrode to the positive left leg lead electrode. The axis of lead III extends from the negative left arm lead electrode to the positive left leg lead electrode.

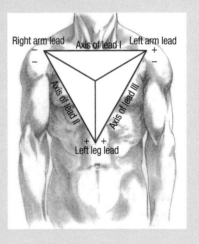

AUGMENTED UNIPOLAR LEADS

Leads aV_R, aV_L, and aV_F are called augmented leads because the small wave-forms that normally would appear from these unipolar leads are enhanced by the ECG.

In lead aV_R, the positive electrode is placed on the right arm and produces a negative deflection because the heart's electrical activity moves away from the lead. In lead aV_L, the positive electrode is on the left arm and usually produces a positive deflection on the ECG. In lead aV_F, the positive electrode is on the left leg (despite the name aV_F) and produces a positive deflection. These three limb leads also provide a view of the heart's frontal plane.

PRECORDIAL UNIPOLAR LEADS

The six unipolar precordial leads are placed in sequence across the chest and provide a view of the heart's horizontal plane. (See *Precordial views*.)

The precordial lead V_1 electrode is placed on the right side of the sternum at the fourth intercostal rib space. This lead shows the P wave, QRS complex, and ST segment particularly well. It helps to distinguish between right and left ventricular ectopic beats that result from myocardial irritation or other cardiac stimulation outside the normal conduction system. Lead V_1 is also useful in monitoring ventricular arrhythmias, ST-segment changes, and bundle-branch blocks.

Augmented unipolar leads

+ Lead aV_R — positive electrode is placed on right arm and produces negative deflection
+ Lead aV_L — positive electrode is placed on left arm and usually produces positive deflection
+ Lead aV_F — positive electrode is placed on left leg and produces positive deflection

Precordial unipolar leads

+ Lead V_1 — placed on right side of sternum at fourth intercostal space (biphasic, with positive and negative deflections)

Precordial views

These illustrations show the different views of the heart obtained from each precordial (chest) lead.

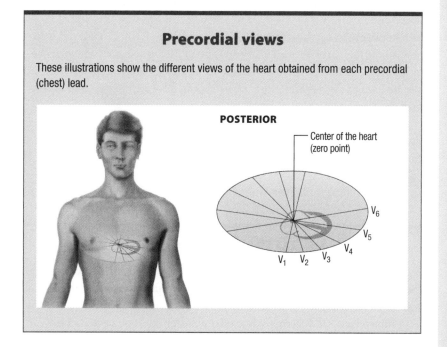

POSTERIOR

Center of the heart (zero point)

V_6
V_5
V_4
V_1 V_2 V_3

Precordial unipolar leads
(continued)

+ Lead V_2 — placed to left of sternum at fourth intercostal space (biphasic, with positive and negative deflections)
+ Lead V_3 — placed between V_2 and V_4 at fifth intercostal space (biphasic, with positive and negative deflections)
+ Lead V_4 — placed at fifth intercostal space at midclavicular line (positive deflection)
+ Lead V_5 — placed between V_4 and V_6 anterior to axillary line (positive deflection)
+ Lead V_6 — placed level with lead V_4 at midaxillary line (positive deflection)

Modified chest leads

+ MCL_1 — negative electrode on left upper chest, positive electrode on right side of heart, and ground electrode on right upper chest
+ MCL_6 — placed at midaxillary line of left fifth intercostal space, negative electrode below left shoulder, and ground below right shoulder

Leadwire systems

+ Three-, four-, or five-electrode system may be used for cardiac monitoring
+ All use ground electrode to prevent accidental electrical shock to patient

Lead V_2 is placed to the left of the sternum at the fourth intercostal space.

Lead V_3 goes between V_2 and V_4 at the fifth intercostal space. Leads V_1, V_2, and V_3 are biphasic, with positive and negative deflections. Leads V_2 and V_3 can be used to detect ST-segment elevation.

Lead V_4 is placed at the fifth intercostal space at the midclavicular line and produces a positive deflection.

Lead V_5 is placed between lead V_4 and V_6 anterior to the axillary line. Lead V_5 produces a positive deflection on the ECG and, along with V_4, can show changes in the ST segment or T wave.

Lead V_6, the last of the precordial leads, is placed level with lead V_4 at the midaxillary line. Lead V_6 produces a positive deflection on the ECG.

MODIFIED CHEST LEADS

MCL stands for modified chest lead. The modification of the chest lead occurs because the actual placement of a negative electrode on the left side of the chest rather than having the center of the heart function as the negative lead. MCL_1 is created by placing the negative electrode on the left upper chest, the positive electrode on the right side of the heart, and the ground electrode usually on the right upper chest. The MCL_1 lead most closely approximates the ECG pattern produced by the chest lead V_1.

When the positive electrode is on the right side of the heart and the electrical current travels toward the left ventricle, the waveform has a negative deflection. As a result, ectopic or abnormal beats deflect in a positive direction.

Choose MCL_1 to assess QRS-complex arrhythmias. You can use this lead to monitor premature ventricular beats and to distinguish different types of tachycardia, such as ventricular and supraventricular tachycardia. MCL_1 can also be used to assess bundle-branch defects and P-wave changes and to confirm pacemaker wire placement.

MCL_6 is an alternative to MCL_1 and most closely approximates the ECG pattern produced by the chest lead V_6. Like MCL_1, it monitors ventricular conduction changes. The positive lead in MCL_6 is placed at the midaxillary line of the left fifth intercostal space, the negative electrode below the left shoulder, and the ground below the right shoulder.

LEADWIRE SYSTEMS

A three-, four-, or five-electrode system may be used for cardiac monitoring. (See *Leadwire systems*.) All three systems use a ground electrode to prevent accidental electrical shock to the patient.

A three-electrode system has one positive electrode, one negative electrode, and a ground. A four-electrode system has a right leg electrode that

Leadwire systems

This chart shows the correct electrode positions for some of the leads you'll use most often — the five-leadwire, three-leadwire, and telemetry systems. The chart uses the abbreviations RA for the right arm, LA for the left arm, RL for the right leg, LL for the left leg, C for the chest, and G for the ground.

ELECTRODE POSITIONS

In the three- and five-leadwire systems, electrode positions for one lead may be identical to those for another lead. When that happens, change the lead selector switch to the setting that corresponds to the lead you want. In some cases, you'll need to reposition the electrodes.

TELEMETRY

In a telemetry monitoring system, you can create the same leads as the other systems with just two electrodes and a ground wire.

Five-leadwire system	**Three-leadwire system**	**Telemetry system**
LEAD I		
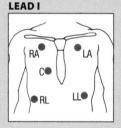	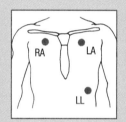	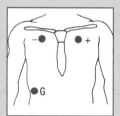
LEAD II		
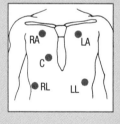	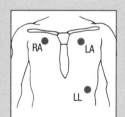	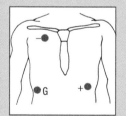
LEAD III		
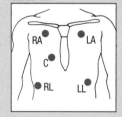	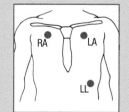	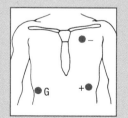

(continued)

Leadwire systems (continued)

Five-leadwire system

LEAD MCL₁

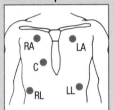

Three-leadwire system

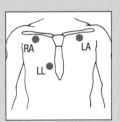

Telemetry system

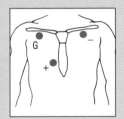

LEAD MCL₆

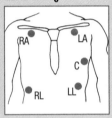

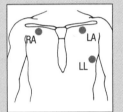

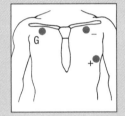

Using a five-leadwire system

This illustration shows the correct placement of the leadwires for a five-leadwire system. The chest electrode shown is located in the lead V_1 position, but you can place it in any of the chest-lead positions. The electrodes are color-coded as follows.

- ✦ White — right arm (RA)
- ✦ Black — left arm (LA)
- ✦ Green — right leg (RL)
- ✦ Red — left leg (LL)
- ✦ Brown — chest (C)

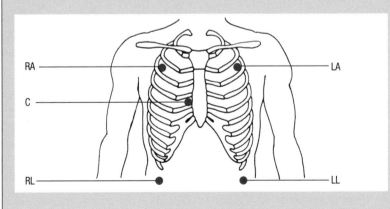

becomes a permanent ground for all leads. The popular five-electrode system is an extension of the four-electrode system and uses an additional exploratory chest lead to allow you to monitor any six modified chest leads as well as the standard limb leads. (See *Using a five-leadwire system.*) This system uses standardized chest placement. Wires that attach to the electrodes are usually color-coded to help you to place them correctly on the patient's chest.

Remember the needs of the patient when applying chest electrodes. For example, if defibrillation is anticipated, avoid placing the electrodes to the right of the sternum and under the left breast, where the paddles would be placed.

APPLICATION OF ELECTRODES

Before attaching electrodes to your patient, make sure he knows you're monitoring his heart rate and rhythm, not controlling them. Tell him not to become upset if he hears an alarm during the procedure; it probably just means a leadwire has come loose.

Explain the electrode placement procedure to the patient, provide privacy, and wash your hands. Expose the patient's chest and select electrode sites for the chosen lead. Choose sites over soft tissues or close to bone, not over bony prominences, thick muscles, or skin folds. Those areas can produce ECG artifacts — waveforms not produced by the heart's electrical activity.

SKIN PREPARATION

Next prepare the patient's skin. Use a special rough patch on the back of the electrode, a dry washcloth, or a gauze pad to briskly rub each site until the skin reddens. Be sure not to damage or break the skin. Brisk scrubbing helps to remove dead skin cells and improves electrical contact.

Hair may interfere with electrical contact; therefore, it may be necessary to clip areas with dense hair. Dry the areas if you moistened them. If the patient has oily skin, clean each site with an alcohol pad and let it air-dry. This ensures proper adhesion and prevents alcohol from becoming trapped beneath the electrode, which can irritate the skin and cause skin breakdown.

APPLICATION OF ELECTRODE PADS

To apply the electrodes, remove the backing and make sure each pregelled electrode is still moist. If an electrode has become dry, discard it and select another. A dry electrode decreases electrical contact and interferes with waveforms.

Apply one electrode to each prepared site using this method:

Application of electrodes
✦ Choose sites over soft tissues or close to bone; not over bony prominences, thick muscles, or skin folds

Skin preparation
✦ Use rough patch on back of electrode, dry washcloth, or gauze pad to rub each site until skin reddens
✦ Clip areas of dense hair (may interfere with electrical contact)
✦ For oily skin, clean each site with alcohol pad, letting it air-dry

Application of electrode pads
✦ Remove backing and make sure each pregelled electrode is still moist
✦ Apply one electrode to each prepared site

◆ Press one side of the electrode against the patient's skin, pull gently, and then press the opposite side of the electrode against the skin.

◆ Using two fingers, press the adhesive edge around the outside of the electrode to the patient's chest. This fixes the gel and stabilizes the electrode.

◆ Repeat this procedure for each electrode.

◆ Every 24 hours, remove the electrodes, assess the patient's skin, and replace the old electrodes with new ones.

Attaching leadwires

◆ Attach leadwires to electrodes

◆ If using snap-on type, attach electrode to leadwire before applying it to patient's chest

◆ If using clip-on leadwire, apply after electrode has been secured to patient's skin

ATTACHING LEADWIRES

You'll also need to attach leadwires, or cable connections, to the monitor. Then, attach leadwires to the electrodes. Leadwires may clip on or, more commonly, snap on. If you're using the snap-on type, attach the electrode to the leadwire before applying it to the patient's chest. You can even do this ahead of time if you know when the patient will arrive. This will help to prevent patient discomfort and disturbances of the contact between the electrode and the skin. When you use a clip-on leadwire, apply it after the electrode has been secured to the patient's skin. That way, applying the clip won't interfere with the electrode's contact with the skin.

Observing cardiac rhythm

◆ Verify that monitor detects each heartbeat by comparing patient's apical rate with rate displayed on monitor

◆ Set upper and lower limits of heart rate per facility policy and patient's condition

◆ Monitors with arrhythmia detection always produce rhythm strip when alarm sounds

◆ Select lead selector button or switch to obtain other views of patient's cardiac rhythm

◆ Press record control on monitor; ECG strip will print at central console (paper consists of horizontal and vertical lines)

OBSERVING CARDIAC RHYTHM

After the electrodes are in proper position, the monitor is on, and the necessary cables are attached, observe the screen. You should see the patient's ECG waveform. Although some monitoring systems allow you to make adjustments by touching the screen, most require you to manipulate knobs and buttons. If the waveform appears too large or too small, change the size by adjusting the gain control. If the waveform appears too high or too low on the screen, adjust the position dial.

Verify that the monitor detects each heartbeat by comparing the patient's apical rate with the rate displayed on the monitor. Set the upper and lower limits of the heart rate according to your facility's policy and the patient's condition. Heart rate alarms are generally set 10 to 20 beats per minute higher or lower than the patient's heart rate.

Monitors with arrhythmia detection generate a rhythm strip automatically whenever the alarm goes off. You can obtain other views of your patient's cardiac rhythm by selecting different leads. You can select leads with the lead selector button or switch.

To get a printout of the patient's cardiac rhythm, press the record control on the monitor. The ECG strip will be printed at the central console. Some systems print the rhythm from a recorder box on the monitor itself.

ECG grid

This electrocardiogram (ECG) grid shows the horizontal axis and vertical axis and their respective measurement values.

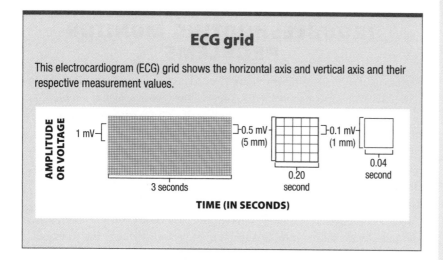

Most monitors can input the patient's name, room number, date, and time as a permanent record; however, if the monitor you're using can't do this, label the rhythm strip with the patient's name, room number, date, time, and rhythm interpretation. Add appropriate clinical information to the ECG strip, such as any medication administered, presence of chest pain, or patient activity at the time of the recording. Be sure to place the rhythm strip in the appropriate section of the patient's medical record.

Waveforms produced by the heart's electrical current are recorded on graphed ECG paper by a heated stylus. ECG paper consists of horizontal and vertical lines forming a grid. A piece of ECG paper is called an *ECG strip* or *tracing*. (See *ECG grid*.)

The horizontal axis of the ECG strip represents time. Each small block equals 0.04 second, and five small blocks form a large block, which equals 0.2 second. This time increment is determined by multiplying 0.04 second (for one small block) by 5, the number of small blocks that compose a large block. Five large blocks equal 1 second (5 × 0.2). When measuring or calculating a patient's heart rate, a 6-second strip consisting of 30 large blocks is usually used.

The ECG strip's vertical axis measures amplitude in millimeters (mm) or electrical voltage in millivolts (mV). Each small block represents 1 mm or 0.1 mV; each large block, 5 mm or 0.5 mV. To determine the amplitude of a wave, segment, or interval, count the number of small blocks from the baseline to the highest or lowest point of the wave, segment, or interval.

Observing cardiac rhythm
(continued)

Horizontal axis
- Represents time
- Each small block equals 0.04 second; five small blocks form large block, equalling 0.2 second
- Time increment is determined by multiplying 0.04 second by 5 (number of small blocks that compose large block)
- Five large blocks equal 1 second (5 × 0.2)
- To calculate patient's heart rate, 6-second strip (30 large blocks) is used

Vertical axis
- Measures amplitude in mm or electrical voltage in mV
- Each small block represents 1 mm or 0.1 mV; each large block, 5 mm or 0.5 mV

Troubleshooting monitor problems

+ *Artifact*—seen with excessive movement; baseline appears wavy, bumpy, or tremulous
+ *Electrical interference*—caused by electrical power leakage
+ *Wandering baseline*—caused by chest wall movement during respiration or poor electrode placement or contact

TROUBLESHOOTING MONITOR PROBLEMS

For optimal cardiac monitoring, you need to recognize problems that can interfere with obtaining a reliable ECG recording. (See *The look of monitor problems.*) Causes of interference include artifact from patient movement and poorly placed or poorly functioning equipment.

Artifact, also called *waveform interference,* may be seen with excessive movement (*somatic tremor*). The baseline of the ECG appears wavy, bumpy, or tremulous. Dry electrodes may also cause this problem due to poor contact.

Electrical interference or AC interference, also called *60-cycle interference,* is caused by electrical power leakage. It may also occur due to interference from other room equipment or improperly grounded equipment. As a result, the lost current pulses at a rate of 60 cycles per second. This interference appears on the ECG as a baseline that is thick and unreadable.

A wandering baseline undulates, meaning that all waveforms are present but the baseline isn't stationary. Movement of the chest wall during respiration, poor electrode placement, or poor electrode contact usually causes this problem.

Faulty equipment, such as broken leadwires and cables, can also cause monitoring problems. Excessively worn equipment can cause improper grounding, putting the patient at risk for accidental shock.

Be aware that some types of artifact resemble arrhythmias and the monitor will interpret them as such. For example, the monitor may sense a small movement, such as the patient brushing his teeth, as a potentially lethal ventricular tachycardia. So, remember to treat the patient, not the monitor. The more familiar you become with your unit's monitoring system—and with your patient—the more quickly you can recognize and interpret problems and act appropriately.

The look of monitor problems

These illustrations present the most commonly encountered monitor problems, including how to identify them, their possible causes, and interventions.

WAVEFORM	POSSIBLE CAUSES	INTERVENTIONS
Artifact (waveform interference)	✦ Patient experiencing seizures, chills, or anxiety	✦ If the patient is having a seizure, notify the physician and intervene as ordered. ✦ Keep the patient warm and encourage him to relax.
	✦ Dirty or corroded connections	✦ Replace dirty or corroded wires.
	✦ Improper electrode application	✦ Check the electrodes and reapply them if needed. Clean the patient's skin well because skin oils and dead skin cells inhibit conduction.
	✦ Dry electrode gel	✦ Check the electrode gel. If the gel is dry, apply new electrodes.
	✦ Short circuit in leadwires or cable	✦ Replace broken equipment.
	✦ Electrical interference from other equipment in the room	✦ Make sure all electrical equipment is attached to a common ground. Check all three-pronged plugs to ensure that none of the prongs are loose. Notify biomedical department.
	✦ Static electricity interference from inadequate room humidity	✦ Regulate room humidity to 40% if possible.
False high-rate alarm	✦ Gain setting too high, particularly with MCL_1 setting	✦ Assess the patient for signs and symptoms of hyperkalemia. ✦ Reset gain.
	✦ HIGH alarm set too low, or LOW alarm set too high	✦ Set alarm limits according to the patient's heart rate.

(continued)

The look of monitor problems *(continued)*

WAVEFORM	POSSIBLE CAUSES	INTERVENTIONS
Weak signals	✦ Improper electrode application	✦ Reapply the electrodes.
	✦ QRS complex too small to register	✦ Reset gain so that the height of the complex is greater than 1 mV. ✦ Try monitoring the patient on another lead.
	✦ Wire or cable failure	✦ Replace any faulty wires or cables.
Wandering baseline	✦ Patient restless	✦ Encourage the patient to relax.
	✦ Chest wall movement during respiration	✦ Make sure that tension on the cable isn't pulling the electrode away from the patient's body.
	✦ Improper electrode application; electrode positioned over bone	✦ Reposition improperly placed electrodes.
Fuzzy baseline (electrical interference)	✦ Electrical interference from other equipment in the room	✦ Ensure that all electrical equipment is attached to a common ground. ✦ Check all three-pronged plugs to make sure none of the prongs are loose.
	✦ Improper grounding of the patient's bed	✦ Ensure that the bed ground is attached to the room's common ground.
	✦ Electrode malfunction	✦ Replace the electrodes.
Baseline (no waveform)	✦ Improper electrode placement (perpendicular to axis of heart)	✦ Reposition improperly placed electrodes.
	✦ Electrode disconnected	✦ Check if electrodes are disconnected.
	✦ Dry electrode gel	✦ Check electrode gel. If the gel is dry, apply new electrodes.
	✦ Wire or cable failure	✦ Replace any faulty wires or cables.

Rhythm strip interpretation

An electrocardiogram (ECG) complex represents the electrical events occurring in one cardiac cycle. A complex consists of five waveforms labeled with the letters P, Q, R, S, and T. The middle three letters—Q, R, and S—are referred to as a unit, the QRS complex. ECG tracings represent the conduction of electrical impulses from the atria to the ventricles. (See *ECG waveform components*.)

ECG waveform components

This illustration shows the components of a normal electrocardiogram (ECG) waveform.

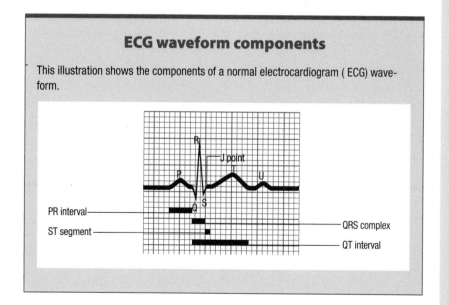

P wave

◆ First component of normal ECG waveform; represents atrial depolarization

◆ If upright in lead II and rounded and smooth, electrical impulse originated in SA node

◆ If peaked, notched, or enlarged, atrial hypertrophy or enlargement

◆ If inverted, retrograde or reverse conduction from AV junction toward atria

◆ If varied, impulse possibly coming from different sites

◆ If absent, possible conduction by a route other than SA node

P WAVE

The P wave is the first component of a normal ECG waveform. It represents atrial depolarization or conduction of an electrical impulse through the atria. When evaluating a P wave, look closely at its characteristics, especially its location, configuration, and deflection. A normal P wave has these characteristics:

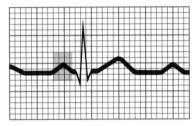

◆ *Location:* precedes the QRS complex
◆ *Amplitude:* 2 to 3 mm high
◆ *Duration:* 0.06 to 0.12 second
◆ *Configuration:* usually rounded and upright
◆ *Deflection:* positive or upright in leads I, II, aV_F, and V_2 to V_6; usually positive but may vary in leads III and aV_L; negative or inverted in lead aV_R; biphasic or variable in lead V_1.

If the deflection and configuration of a P wave are normal — for example, if the P wave is upright in lead II and is rounded and smooth — and if the P wave precedes each QRS complex, you can assume that this electrical impulse originated in the sinoatrial (SA) node. The atria start to contract partway through the P wave, but you won't see this on the ECG. Remember, the ECG records electrical activity only, not mechanical activity or contraction.

Peaked, notched, or enlarged P waves may represent atrial hypertrophy or enlargement associated with chronic obstructive pulmonary disease, pulmonary emboli, valvular disease, or heart failure. Inverted P waves may signify retrograde or reverse conduction from the atrioventricular junction toward the atria. Whenever an upright sinus P wave becomes inverted, consider retrograde or reverse conduction as possible conditions.

Varying P waves indicate that the impulse may be coming from different sites, as with a wandering pacemaker rhythm, irritable atrial tissue, or damage near the SA node. Absent P waves may signify conduction by a route other than the SA node, as with a junctional or atrial fibrillation rhythm. When a P wave doesn't precede the QRS complex, complete heart block may be present.

PR interval

◆ Tracks atrial impulse from atria to AV node, bundle of His, and right and left bundle branches

PR INTERVAL

The PR interval tracks the atrial impulse from the atria through the atrioventricular (AV) node, bundle of His, and right and left bundle branches. When evaluating a PR interval, look especially at its duration. Changes in the PR interval indicate an altered impulse formation or a conduction delay, as seen in AV block. A normal PR interval has these characteristics (amplitude, configuration, and deflection aren't measured):

✦ *Location*: from the beginning of the
P wave to the beginning of the QRS
complex

✦ *Duration:* 0.12 to 0.20 second.
    Short PR intervals (less than
0.12 second) indicate that the impulse
originated somewhere other than the
sinoatrial node. This variation is associ-

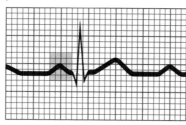

ated with junctional arrhythmias and preexcitation syndromes. Prolonged PR intervals (greater than 0.20 second) may represent a conduction delay through the atria or AV junction due to digoxin toxicity or heart block — slowing related to ischemia or conduction tissue disease.

QRS COMPLEX

The QRS complex follows the P wave and represents depolarization of the ventricles, or impulse conduction. Immediately after the ventricles depolarize, as represented by the QRS complex, they contract. That contraction ejects blood from the ventricles and pumps it through the arteries, creating a pulse.

Whenever you're monitoring cardiac rhythm, remember that the waveform you see represents the heart's electrical activity only. It doesn't guarantee a mechanical contraction of the heart and a subsequent pulse. The contraction could be weak, as happens with premature ventricular contractions, or absent, as happens with pulseless electrical activity. So, before you treat the strip, check the patient.

Pay special attention to the duration and configuration when evaluating a QRS complex. A normal complex has these characteristics:

✦ *Location:* follows the PR interval

✦ *Amplitude:* 5 to 30 mm high, but differs for each lead used

✦ *Duration:* 0.06 to 0.10 second, or half
of the PR interval. Duration is measured from the beginning of the Q wave
to the end of the S wave or from the beginning of the R wave if the Q wave is
absent.

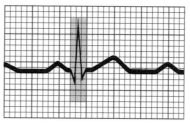

✦ *Configuration:* consists of the Q wave (the first negative deflection, or deflection below the baseline, after the P wave), the R wave (the first positive deflection after the Q wave), and the S wave (the first negative deflection af-

QRS waveform variety

These illustrations show the various configurations of QRS complexes. When documenting the QRS complex, use uppercase letters to indicate a wave with a normal or high amplitude (greater than 5 mm) and lowercase letters to indicate one with a low amplitude (less than 5 mm).

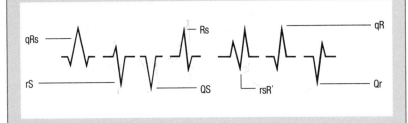

ter the R wave). You may not always see all three waves. The ventricles depolarize quickly, minimizing contact time between the stylus and the ECG paper, so the QRS complex typically appears thinner than other ECG components. It may also look different in each lead. (See *QRS waveform variety*.)

◆ *Deflection*: positive (with most of the complex above the baseline) in leads I, II, III, aV_L, aV_F, and V_4 to V_6, negative in leads aV_R and V_1 to V_2, and biphasic in lead V_3.

Remember that the QRS complex represents intraventricular conduction time. That's why identifying and correctly interpreting it is so crucial. If no P wave appears with the QRS complex, then the impulse may have originated in the ventricles, indicating a ventricular arrhythmia.

Deep, wide Q waves may represent myocardial infarction. In this case, the Q wave amplitude (depth) is greater than or equal to 25% of the height of the succeeding R wave, or the duration of the Q wave is 0.04 second or more. A notched R wave may signify a bundle-branch block. A widened QRS complex (greater than 0.12 second) may signify a ventricular conduction delay. A missing QRS complex may indicate atrioventricular block or ventricular standstill.

QRS complex
(continued)
◆ Widened QRS complex (> 0.12 second) may signify ventricular conduction delay
◆ Missing QRS complex may indicate AV block or ventricular standstill

ST segment
◆ Represents end of ventricular depolarization and onset of ventricular repolarization

ST SEGMENT

The ST segment represents the end of ventricular conduction or depolarization and the beginning of ventricular recovery or repolarization. The point that marks the end of the QRS complex and the beginning of the ST segment is known as the *J point.*

Pay special attention to the deflection of an ST segment. A normal ST segment has these characteristics (amplitude, duration, and configuration aren't observed):

✦ *Location:* extends from the S wave to the beginning of the T wave

✦ *Deflection:* usually isoelectric (neither positive nor negative); may vary from −0.5 to +1 mm in some precordial leads.

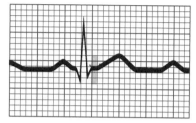

A change in the ST segment may indicate myocardial injury or ischemia. An ST segment may become either elevated or depressed. (See *Changes in the ST segment.*)

Changes in the ST segment

Closely monitoring the ST segment on a patient's electrocardiogram can help you detect ischemia or injury before infarction develops.

ST-SEGMENT DEPRESSION
An ST segment is considered depressed when it's 0.5 mm or more below the baseline. A depressed ST segment may indicate myocardial ischemia or digoxin toxicity.

ST-SEGMENT ELEVATION
An ST segment is considered elevated when it's 1 mm or more above the baseline. An elevated ST segment may indicate myocardial injury.

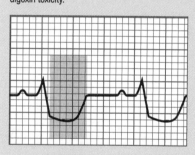
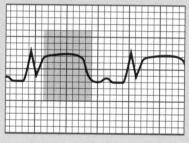

T WAVE

The peak of the T wave represents the relative refractory period of repolarization or ventricular recovery. When evaluating a T wave, look at the amplitude, configuration, and deflection.

T wave
(continued)

Normal T wave
+ *Location*—follows ST segment
+ *Configuration*—typically rounded and smooth
+ Bumps may indicate embedded P wave
+ If tall, peaked, or tented, possible myocardial injury or electrolyte imbalances (hyperkalemia)
+ If inverted, possible myocardial ischemia

Normal T waves have these characteristics (duration isn't measured):
+ *Location:* follows the ST segment
+ *Amplitude:* 0.5 mm in leads I, II, and III and up to 10 mm in the precordial leads
+ *Configuration:* typically rounded and smooth
+ *Deflection:* usually positive or upright in leads I, II, and V_2 to V_6; inverted in lead aV_R; variable leads III and V_1.

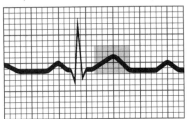

The T wave's peak represents the relative refractory period of ventricular repolarization, a period during which cells are especially vulnerable to extra stimuli. Bumps in a T wave may indicate that a P wave is hidden in it. If a P wave is hidden, atrial depolarization has occurred, the impulse having originated at a site above the ventricles.

Tall, peaked, or "tented" T waves may indicate myocardial injury or electrolyte imbalances such as hyperkalemia. Inverted T waves in leads I, II, aV_L, aV_F, or V_2 through V_6 may represent myocardial ischemia. Heavily notched or pointed T waves in an adult may indicate pericarditis.

QT interval
+ Measures time needed for ventricular depolarization and repolarization
+ Length varies according to heart rate

Normal QT interval
+ *Location*—extends from beginning of QRS complex to end of T wave
+ *Duration*—usually lasts from 0.36 to 0.44 second
+ Prolonged QT intervals indicate slowed ventricular repolarization; also associated with medications (class I antiarrhythmics)
+ Short QT intervals may result from digoxin toxicity or electrolyte imbalances (hypercalcemia)

QT INTERVAL

The QT interval measures the time needed for ventricular depolarization and repolarization. The length of the QT interval varies according to heart rate. The faster the heart rate, the shorter the QT interval. When checking the QT interval, look closely at the duration.

A normal QT interval has these characteristics (amplitude, configuration, and deflection aren't observed):
+ *Location:* extends from the beginning of the QRS complex to the end of the T wave
+ *Duration:* varies according to age, sex, and heart rate; usually lasts from 0.36 to 0.44 second; shouldn't be greater than half the distance between the two consecutive R waves (called the *R-R interval*) when the rhythm is regular.

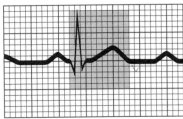

The QT interval measures the time needed for ventricular depolarization and repolarization. Prolonged QT intervals indicate that ventricular repolarization time is slowed, meaning that the relative refractory or vulnerable period of the cardiac cycle is longer.

This variation is also associated with certain medications such as class I antiarrhythmics. Prolonged QT syndrome is a congenital conduction-system defect present in certain families. Short QT intervals may result from digoxin toxicity or electrolyte imbalances such as hypercalcemia.

U WAVE

The U wave represents repolarization of the His-Purkinje system or ventricular conduction fibers. It isn't present on every rhythm strip. The configuration is the most important characteristic of the U wave.

When present, a normal U wave has these characteristics (amplitude and duration aren't measured):
+ *Location*: follows the T wave
+ *Configuration*: typically upright and rounded
+ *Deflection*: upright.

The U wave may not appear on an ECG. A prominent U wave may be due to hypercalcemia, hypokalemia, or digoxin toxicity.

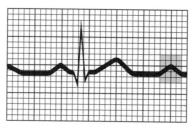

NORMAL SINUS RHYTHM

Before you can recognize an arrhythmia, you first need to be able to recognize a normal cardiac rhythm. The term *arrhythmia* literally means an absence of rhythm. The more accurate term dysrhythmia means an abnormality in rhythm. These terms, however, are frequently used interchangeably.

Normal sinus rhythm (NSR) occurs when an impulse starts in the sinus node and progresses to the ventricles through a normal conduction pathway—from the sinus node to the atria and atrioventricular node, through the bundle of His, to the bundle branches, and on to the Purkinje fibers. There are no premature or aberrant contractions. NSR is the standard against which all other rhythms are compared. (*See Recognizing normal sinus rhythm*, page 42.)

Practice the eight-step method, described below, to analyze an ECG strip with a normal cardiac rhythm, known as NSR. The ECG characteristics of NSR include:
+ *Rhythm*: atrial and ventricular rhythms are regular
+ *Rate:* atrial and ventricular rates are 60 to 100 beats/minute, the sinoatrial node's normal firing rate
+ *P wave*: normally shaped (round and smooth) and upright in lead II; all P waves similar in size and shape; a P wave for every QRS complex

---

U wave
+ Represents repolarization of His-Purkinje system

Normal U wave
+ *Location*—follows T wave
+ *Configuration*—typically upright and rounded
+ If prominent, possible hypercalcemia, hypokalemia, or digoxin toxicity

Normal sinus rhythm
+ Impulse starts in sinus node, progressing to ventricles through normal conduction pathway
+ Standard against which all rhythms are compared

NSR characteristics
+ *Rhythm*—atrial and ventricular rhythms regular
+ *Rate*—60 to 100 beats/minute
+ *P wave*—normally shaped
+ *PR interval*—within normal limits

Recognizing normal sinus rhythm

Normal sinus rhythm, shown below, represents normal impulse conduction through the heart.

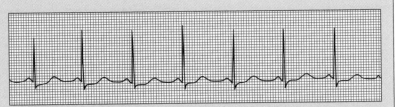

◆ *Rhythm:* atrial and ventricular rhythms regular
◆ *Rate:* atrial and ventricular rates normal; 60 beats/minute
◆ *P wave:* normal; precedes each QRS complex; all P waves similar in size and shape

◆ *PR interval:* normal; 0.10 second
◆ *QRS complex:* 0.06 second
◆ *T wave:* normal shape (upright and rounded)
◆ *QT interval:* normal; 0.40 second
◆ *Other:* no ectopic or aberrantly conducted impulses

Normal sinus rhythm
(continued)

NSR characteristics
◆ *QRS complex*—within normal limits
◆ *T wave*—normally shaped
◆ *QT interval*—within normal limits
◆ *Other*—no ectopic or aberrant beats

◆ *PR interval:* within normal limits (0.12 to 0.20 second)
◆ *QRS complex:* within normal limits (0.06 to 0.10 second)
◆ *T wave:* normally shaped; upright and rounded in lead II
◆ *QT interval:* within normal limits (0.36 to 0.44 second)
◆ *Other:* no ectopic or aberrant beats. (See *ECG changes in the older adult.*)

AGE CHANGE

ECG changes in the older adult

Always keep the patient's age in mind when interpreting the electrocardiogram (ECG). Changes that might be seen in the ECG of an older adult include increased PR, QRS, and QT intervals, decreased amplitude of the QRS complex, and a shift of the QRS axis to the left.

THE 8-STEP METHOD

Analyzing a rhythm strip is a skill developed through practice. You can use several methods, as long as you're consistent. Rhythm strip analysis requires a sequential and systematic approach such as the eight steps outlined here.

STEP 1: DETERMINE RHYTHM

To determine the heart's atrial and ventricular rhythms, use either the paper-and-pencil method or the caliper method. (See *Methods of measuring rhythm*, page 44.)

For atrial rhythm, measure the P-P intervals; that is, the intervals between consecutive P waves. These intervals should occur regularly, with only small variations associated with respirations. Then compare the P-P intervals in several cycles. Consistently similar P-P intervals indicate regular atrial rhythm; dissimilar P-P intervals indicate irregular atrial rhythm.

To determine the ventricular rhythm, measure the intervals between two consecutive R waves in the QRS complexes. If an R wave isn't present, use either the Q wave or the S wave of consecutive QRS complexes. The R-R intervals should occur regularly. Then compare R-R intervals in several cycles. As with atrial rhythms, consistently similar intervals mean a regular rhythm; dissimilar intervals point to an irregular rhythm.

After completing your measurements, ask yourself:
✦ Is the rhythm regular or irregular? Consider a rhythm with only slight variations, up to 0.04 second, to be regular.
✦ If the rhythm is irregular, is it slightly irregular or markedly so? Does the irregularity occur in a pattern (a regularly irregular pattern)?

STEP 2: CALCULATE RATE

You can use one of three methods to determine atrial and ventricular heart rates from an ECG waveform. Although these methods can provide accurate information, you shouldn't rely solely on them when assessing your patient. Keep in mind that the ECG waveform represents electrical, not mechanical, activity. Therefore, although an ECG can show you that ventricular depolarization has occurred, it doesn't mean that ventricular contraction has occurred. To do this, you must assess the patient's pulse. So remember, always check a pulse to correlate it with the heart rate on the ECG.
✦ Times-ten method. The simplest, quickest, and most common way to calculate rate is the times ten method, especially if the rhythm is irregular. ECG paper is marked in increments of 3 seconds, or 15 large boxes. To calculate the atrial rate, obtain a 6-second strip, count the number of P waves on it,

The 8-step method
✦ Rhythm strip analysis requires sequential and systematic approach

Step 1: Determine rhythm
✦ Use paper-and-pencil method or caliper method
✦ *Atrial rhythm*—measure P-P intervals
✦ *Ventricular rhythm*—measure intervals between two consecutive R waves in QRS complexes
After completing measurements, ask yourself:
✦ Is rhythm regular or irregular?
✦ If irregular, is it only slightly or markedly so?

Step 2: Calculate rate
✦ Use one of three methods to determine atrial and ventricular heart rates
✦ *Times-ten method*—simplest, quickest, and most common

KNOW-HOW

Methods of measuring rhythm

You can use either of these methods to determine atrial or ventricular rhythm.

PAPER-AND-PENCIL METHOD

Place the ECG strip on a flat surface. Then position the straight edge of a piece of paper along the strip's baseline. Move the paper up slightly so the straight edge is near the peak of the R wave.

With a pencil, mark the paper at the R waves of two consecutive QRS complexes, as shown above. This is the R-R interval. Next, move the paper across the strip lining up the two marks with succeeding R-R intervals. If the distance for each R-R interval is the same, the ventricular rhythm is regular. If the distance varies, the rhythm is irregular.

Use the same method to measure the distance between the P waves (the P-P interval) and determine whether the atrial rhythm is regular or irregular.

CALIPER METHOD

With the ECG on a flat surface, place one point of the calipers on the peak of the first R wave of two consecutive QRS complexes. Then adjust the caliper legs so the other point is on the peak of the next R wave, as shown above. This distance is the R-R interval.

Now pivot the first point of the calipers toward the third R wave and note whether it falls on the peak of that wave. Check succeeding R-R intervals in the same way. If they're all the same, the ventricular rhythm is regular. If they vary, the rhythm is irregular.

Using the same method, measure the P-P intervals to determine whether the atrial rhythm is regular or irregular.

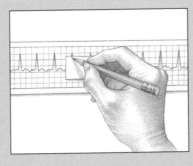
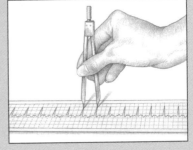

Step 2: Calculate rate
(continued)

+ *1,500 method*—if heart rhythm is regular
+ *Sequence method*—requires memorizing sequence of numbers (300, 150, 100, 75, 60, 50)

and multiply by 10. Ten 6-second strips equal 1 minute. Calculate ventricular rate the same way, using the R waves.

+ 1,500 method. If the heart rhythm is regular, use the 1,500 method, so named because 1,500 small squares equals 1 minute. Count the number of small squares between identical points on two consecutive P waves, and then divide 1,500 by that number to get the atrial rate. To obtain the ventricular rate, use the same method with two consecutive R waves.

✦ Sequence method. The third method of estimating heart rate is the sequence method, which requires memorizing a sequence of numbers. For atrial rate, find a P wave that peaks on a heavy black line and assign the following numbers to the next six heavy black lines: 300, 150, 100, 75, 60, and 50. Then find the next P wave peak and estimate the atrial rate, based on the number assigned to the nearest heavy black line. Estimate the ventricular rate the same way, using the R wave.

STEP 3: EVALUATE P WAVE

When examining a rhythm strip for P waves, ask yourself:
✦ Are P waves present?
✦ Do the P waves have a normal configuration?
✦ Do all the P waves have a similar size and shape?
✦ Is there one P wave for every QRS complex?

STEP 4: DETERMINE PR INTERVAL DURATION

To measure the PR interval, count the small squares between the start of the P wave and the start of the QRS complex; then multiply the number of squares by 0.04 second. After performing this calculation, ask yourself:
✦ Does the duration of the PR interval fall within normal limits, 0.12 to 0.20 second (or 3 to 5 small squares)?
✦ Is the PR interval constant?

STEP 5: DETERMINE QRS COMPLEX DURATION

When determining QRS complex duration, make sure you measure straight across from the end of the PR interval to the end of the S wave, not just to the peak. Remember, the QRS complex has no horizontal components. To calculate duration, count the number of small squares between the beginning and end of the QRS complex and multiply this number by 0.04 second. Then ask yourself:
✦ Does the duration of the QRS complex fall within normal limits, 0.06 to 0.10 second?
✦ Are all QRS complexes the same size and shape? (If not, measure each one and describe them individually.)
✦ Does a QRS complex appear after every P wave?

STEP 6: EVALUATE T WAVE

Examine the T waves on the ECG strip. Then ask yourself:
✦ Are T waves present?
✦ Do all of the T waves have a normal shape?

Step 3: Evaluate P wave
After examining strip, ask yourself:
✦ Are they present?
✦ Normal configuration?
✦ Similar size and shape?
✦ One for every QRS complex?

Step 4: Determine PR interval duration
After performing calculation, ask yourself:
✦ Fall within normal limits (0.12 to 0.20 second)?
✦ Is it constant?

Step 5: Determine QRS complex duration
After performing calculation, ask yourself:
✦ Fall within normal limits (0.06 to 0.10 second)?
✦ Same size and shape?
✦ Appear after every P wave?

Step 6: Evaluate T wave
After examining strip, ask yourself:
✦ Are they present?
✦ Normal shape?

Step 6: Evaluate T wave
(continued)
+ Could P wave be hidden within?
+ Normal amplitude?
+ Same deflection as QRS complexes?

Step 7: Determine QT interval duration
After performing calculation, ask yourself:
+ Fall within normal limits (0.36 to 0.44 second)?

Step 8: Evaluate other components
+ Note presence of ectopic or aberrantly conducted beats or other abnormalities
+ Check ST segment for abnormalities; look for U wave

+ Could a P wave be hidden in a T wave?
+ Do all T waves have a normal amplitude?
+ Do the T waves have the same deflection as the QRS complexes?

STEP 7: DETERMINE QT INTERVAL DURATION

Count the number of small squares between the beginning of the QRS complex and the end of the T wave, where the T wave returns to the baseline. Multiply this number by 0.04 second. Ask yourself:
+ Does the duration of the QT interval fall within normal limits, 0.36 to 0.44 second?

STEP 8: EVALUATE OTHER COMPONENTS

Note the presence of ectopic or aberrantly conducted beats or other abnormalities. Also check the ST segment for abnormalities, and look for the presence of a U wave.

Now, interpret your findings by classifying the rhythm strip according to one or all of the following:
+ *Site of origin of the rhythm*: for example, sinus node, atria, atrioventricular node, or ventricles
+ *Rate*: normal (60 to 100 beats/minute), bradycardia (less than 60 beats/minute), or tachycardia (greater than 100 beats/minute) (See *Pediatric rates and intervals*.)
+ *Rhythm*: normal or abnormal; for example, flutter, fibrillation, heart block, escape rhythm, or other arrhythmias.

AGE CHANGE

Pediatric rates and intervals

The hearts of infants and children beat faster than those of adults because children have smaller ventricular size and higher metabolic needs. The fast heart rate and small size produce short PR intervals and QRS duration.

Age	Heart rate (beats/min)	PR interval (second)	QRS duration (second)
1 to 3 weeks	100 to 180	0.07 to 0.14	0.03 to 0.07
1 to 6 months	100 to 185	0.07 to 0.16	0.03 to 0.07
7 to 11 months	100 to 170	0.08 to 0.16	0.03 to 0.08
1 to 3 years	90 to 150	0.09 to 0.16	0.03 to 0.08
4 to 5 years	70 to 140	0.09 to 0.16	0.03 to 0.08
6 to 7 years	65 to 130	0.09 to 0.16	0.03 to 0.08
8 to 11 years	60 to 110	0.09 to 0.16	0.03 to 0.09
12 to 16 years	60 to 100	0.09 to 0.18	0.03 to 0.09

Sinus node arrhythmias

When the heart functions normally, the sinoatrial (SA) node, also called the *sinus node,* acts as the primary pacemaker. The sinus node assumes this role because its automatic firing rate exceeds that of the heart's other pacemakers. In an adult at rest, the sinus node has an inherent firing rate of 60 to 100 times per minute.

In approximately 50% of the population, the SA node's blood supply comes from the right coronary artery, and from the left circumflex artery in the other half of the population. The autonomic nervous system (ANS) richly innervates the sinus node through the vagal nerve, a parasympathetic nerve, and several sympathetic nerves. Stimulation of the vagus nerve decreases the node's firing rate, and stimulation of the sympathetic system increases it.

Changes in the automaticity of the sinus node, alterations in its blood supply, and ANS influences may all lead to sinus node arrhythmias. This chapter will help you to identify sinus node arrhythmias on an electrocardiogram (ECG). It will also help you to determine the causes, clinical significance, signs and symptoms, and interventions associated with each arrhythmia presented.

The 8-step method to analyze the ECG strip will be used for each of the following arrhythmias.

Sinus arrhythmia

✦ Rate stays within normal limits; but, rhythm is irregular and corresponds to respiratory cycle

Causes

✦ Results from inhibition of reflex vagal activity, or tone
✦ Other causes: heart disease, inferior wall MI, and certain drugs (digoxin, morphine)

SINUS ARRHYTHMIA

In sinus tachycardia and sinus bradycardia, the cardiac rate falls outside the normal limits. In sinus arrhythmia, the rate stays within normal limits but the rhythm is irregular and corresponds to the respiratory cycle. Sinus arrhythmia can occur normally in athletes, children, and older adults, but it rarely occurs in infants.

CAUSES

Sinus arrhythmia, the heart's normal response to respirations, results from an inhibition of reflex vagal activity, or tone. During inspiration, an increase in the flow of blood back to the heart reduces vagal tone, which increases the heart rate. ECG complexes fall closer together, which shortens the P-P interval. During expiration, venous return decreases, which in turn increases vagal tone, slows the heart rate, and lengthens the P-P interval. (See *Recognizing sinus arrhythmia.*)

Conditions unrelated to respiration may also produce sinus arrhythmia, including heart disease; inferior wall myocardial infarction; the use of certain drugs, such as digoxin and morphine; and conditions involving increased intracranial pressure.

CLINICAL SIGNIFICANCE

Sinus arrhythmia usually isn't significant and produces no symptoms. A marked variation in P-P intervals in an older adult, however, may indicate sick sinus syndrome — a related, but potentially more serious, phenomenon.

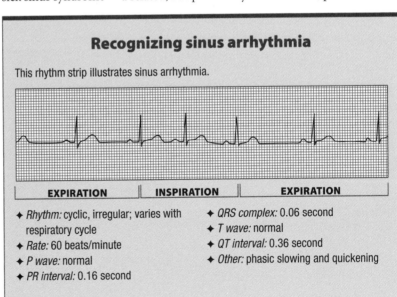

Recognizing sinus arrhythmia

This rhythm strip illustrates sinus arrhythmia.

EXPIRATION | INSPIRATION | EXPIRATION

✦ *Rhythm:* cyclic, irregular; varies with respiratory cycle
✦ *Rate:* 60 beats/minute
✦ *P wave:* normal
✦ *PR interval:* 0.16 second
✦ *QRS complex:* 0.06 second
✦ *T wave:* normal
✦ *QT interval:* 0.36 second
✦ *Other:* phasic slowing and quickening

ECG CHARACTERISTICS

✦ *Rhythm:* Atrial rhythm is irregular, corresponding to the respiratory cycle. The P-P interval is shorter during inspiration, longer during expiration. The difference between the longest and shortest P-P interval exceeds 0.12 second. Ventricular rhythm is also irregular, corresponding to the respiratory cycle. The R-R interval is shorter during inspiration, longer during expiration. The difference between the longest and shortest R-R interval exceeds 0.12 second.

✦ *Rate:* Atrial and ventricular rates are within normal limits (60 to 100 beats/ minute) and vary with respiration. Typically, the heart rate increases during inspiration and decreases during expiration.

✦ *P wave:* Normal size and configuration; P wave precedes each QRS complex.

✦ *PR interval:* May vary slightly within normal limits.

✦ *QRS complex:* Normal duration and configuration.

✦ *QT wave:* Normal size and configuration.

✦ *QT interval:* May vary slightly, but usually within normal limits.

✦ *Other:* None.

SIGNS AND SYMPTOMS

The patient's peripheral pulse rate increases during inspiration and decreases during expiration. Sinus arrhythmia is easier to detect when the heart rate is slow; it may disappear when the heart rate increases, as with exercise.

If the arrhythmia is caused by an underlying condition, you may note signs and symptoms of that condition. Marked sinus arrhythmia may cause dizziness or syncope in some cases.

INTERVENTIONS

Unless the patient is symptomatic, treatment usually isn't necessary. If sinus arrhythmia is unrelated to respirations, the underlying cause may require treatment.

When caring for a patient with sinus arrhythmia, observe the heart rhythm during respiration to determine whether the arrhythmia coincides with the respiratory cycle. Be sure to check the monitor carefully to avoid an inaccurate interpretation of the waveform.

If sinus arrhythmia is induced by drugs, such as morphine and other sedatives, the physician may decide to continue to give the patient those medications. If sinus arrhythmia develops suddenly in a patient taking digoxin, notify the physician immediately. The patient may be experiencing digoxin toxicity.

ECG characteristics

✦ *Rhythm*—atrial and ventricular rhythm irregular, corresponding to respiratory cycle
✦ *Rate*—atrial and ventricular rates within normal limits; vary with respiration
✦ *P wave*—normal size and configuration
✦ *PR interval*—may vary (slightly) within normal limits
✦ *QRS complex*—normal duration and configuration

Signs and symptoms

✦ Peripheral pulse rate increases during inspiration; decreases during expiration
✦ If caused by underlying condition, signs and symptoms of that condition
✦ Possible dizziness or syncope

Interventions

✦ Unnecessary in asymptomatic patient
✦ If unrelated to respirations, treat underlying cause

Sinus bradycardia

+ Sinus rate below 60 beats/minute and regular rhythm
+ Impulses originate in SA node

Causes

+ Increased intracranial pressure
+ Hypothyroidism
+ Hypothermia
+ Glaucoma
+ Cardiac diseases (SA node disease, cardiomyopathy, myocardial ischemia)
+ Drugs (beta-adrenergic blockers, digoxin, calcium channel blockers)
+ *Note:* May occur normally during sleep or in person with well-conditioned heart (athlete)

SINUS BRADYCARDIA

Sinus bradycardia is characterized by a sinus rate below 60 beats/minute and a regular rhythm. All impulses originate in the sinoatrial node (SA) node. This arrhythmia's significance depends on the symptoms and the underlying cause. Unless the patient shows symptoms of decreased cardiac output, no treatment is necessary. (See *Recognizing sinus bradycardia* and *Bradycardia and tachycardia in children*.)

CAUSES

Sinus bradycardia usually occurs as the normal response to a reduced demand for blood flow. In this case, vagal stimulation increases and sympathetic stimulation decreases. As a result, *automaticity* (the tendency of cells to initiate their own impulses) in the SA node diminishes. It may occur normally during sleep or in a person with a well-conditioned heart—an athlete, for example.

Sinus bradycardia may be caused by:

+ noncardiac disorders, such as hyperkalemia, increased intracranial pressure, hypothyroidism, hypothermia, and glaucoma
+ conditions producing excess vagal stimulation or decreased sympathetic stimulation, such as sleep, deep relaxation, Valsalva's maneuver, carotid sinus massage, and vomiting
+ cardiac diseases, such as SA node disease, cardiomyopathy, myocarditis, and myocardial ischemia; can also occur immediately following an inferior

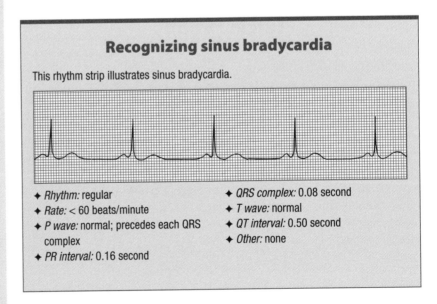

Recognizing sinus bradycardia

This rhythm strip illustrates sinus bradycardia.

+ *Rhythm:* regular
+ *Rate:* < 60 beats/minute
+ *P wave:* normal; precedes each QRS complex
+ *PR interval:* 0.16 second
+ *QRS complex:* 0.08 second
+ *T wave:* normal
+ *QT interval:* 0.50 second
+ *Other:* none

Bradycardia and tachycardia in children

Evaluate bradycardia and tachycardia in children in context. Bradycardia (less than 90 beats/minute) may occur in the healthy infant during sleep, and tachycardia may occur when the child is crying or otherwise upset. Because the heart rate varies considerably from the neonate to the adolescent, neither bradycardia nor tachycardia can be assigned a single definition to be used for all children.

wall myocardial infarction (MI) that involves the right coronary artery, which supplies blood to the SA node

✦ certain drugs, especially beta-adrenergic blockers, digoxin, calcium channel blockers, lithium, and antiarrhythmics, such as sotalol, amiodarone, propafenone, and quinidine.

CLINICAL SIGNIFICANCE

The clinical significance of sinus bradycardia depends on how low the rate is and whether the patient is symptomatic. For example, most adults can tolerate a sinus bradycardia of 45 to 59 beats/minute but are less tolerant of a rate below 45 beats/minute.

Usually, sinus bradycardia produces symptoms and is insignificant. Many athletes develop sinus bradycardia because their well-conditioned hearts can maintain a normal stroke volume with less-than-normal effort. Sinus bradycardia also occurs normally during sleep as a result of circadian variations in heart rate.

When sinus bradycardia produces no symptoms, however, prompt attention is critical. The heart of a patient with underlying cardiac disease may not be able to compensate for a drop in rate by increasing its stroke volume. The resulting drop in cardiac output produces such signs and symptoms as hypotension and dizziness. Bradycardia may also predispose some patients to more serious arrhythmias, such as ventricular tachycardia and ventricular fibrillation.

In a patient with acute inferior wall MI, sinus bradycardia is considered a favorable prognostic sign, unless it's accompanied by hypotension. Because sinus bradycardia rarely affects children, it's considered a poor prognostic sign in ill children.

ECG CHARACTERISTICS

✦ *Rhythm:* Atrial and ventricular rhythms are regular.

ECG characteristics
✦ *Rhythm*—atrial and ventricular rhythms regular

ECG characteristics
(continued)

+ *Rate* — atrial and ventricular rates < 60 beats/minute
+ *P wave* — normal size and configuration
+ *PR interval* — within normal limits and constant
+ *QRS complex* — normal duration and configuration
+ *QT interval* — within normal limits, but may be prolonged

Signs and symptoms

+ Pulse rate < 60 beats/minute; usually asymptomatic

If compensatory mechanisms fail
+ Hypotension
+ Cool, clammy skin
+ Altered mental status
+ Dizziness
+ Blurred vision
+ Crackles, dyspnea, and S₃ (heart failure)
+ Chest pain
+ Syncope

Interventions

+ Unnecessary in asymptomatic patient (with stable vital signs)
+ If symptomatic, identify and correct underlying cause

+ *Rate:* Atrial and ventricular rates are less than 60 beats/minute.
+ *P wave:* Normal size and configuration; P wave precedes each QRS complex.
+ *PR interval:* Within normal limits and constant.
+ *QRS complex:* Normal duration and configuration.
+ *T wave:* Normal size and configuration.
+ *QT interval:* Within normal limits, but may be prolonged.
+ *Other:* None.

SIGNS AND SYMPTOMS

The patient will have a pulse rate of less than 60 beats/minute, with a regular rhythm. As long as he's able to compensate for the decreased cardiac output, he's likely to remain asymptomatic. If compensatory mechanisms fail, however, signs and symptoms of declining cardiac output usually appear, including:

+ hypotension
+ cool, clammy skin
+ altered mental status
+ dizziness
+ blurred vision
+ crackles, dyspnea, and an S_3 heart sound, indicating heart failure
+ chest pain
+ syncope.

   Palpitations and pulse irregularities may occur if the patient experiences ectopy such as premature atrial, junctional, or ventricular contractions. This is because the SA node's increased relative refractory period permits ectopic firing. Bradycardia-induced syncope (Stokes-Adams attack) may also occur.

INTERVENTIONS

If the patient is asymptomatic and his vital signs are stable, treatment generally isn't necessary. Continue to observe his heart rhythm, monitoring the progression and duration of the bradycardia. Evaluate his tolerance of the rhythm at rest and with activity. Review the medications he's taking. Check with the physician about stopping medications that may be depressing the SA node, such as digoxin, beta-adrenergic blockers, or calcium channel blockers. Before giving these drugs, make sure the heart rate is within a safe range.

   If the patient is symptomatic, treatment aims to identify and correct the underlying cause. Meanwhile, the heart rate must be maintained with such drugs as atropine, dopamine, and epinephrine or with a transvenous or transcutaneous pacemaker. (See *Bradycardia algorithm.*) Keep in mind that a patient with a transplanted heart won't respond to atropine and may require

Bradycardia algorithm

A patient with a bradycardic rhythm may either show few symptoms or show symptoms of decreased cardiac output. If the patient does have decreased cardiac output, determine the cause and initiate appropriate treatments.

Bradycardia
- ◆ Slow (absolute bradycardia = rate < 60 beats/minute)

   or
- ◆ Relatively slow (rate less than expected relative to underlying condition or cause)

Primary ABCD survey
- ◆ Assess ABCs.
- ◆ Secure airway noninvasively.
- ◆ Ensure monitor or defibrillator is available.

Secondary ABCD survey
- ◆ Assess secondary ABCs. (Invasive airway management needed?)
- ◆ Apply oxygen; establish I.V. access; monitor; administer fluids.
- ◆ Monitor vital signs, pulse oximetry, blood pressure.
- ◆ Obtain and review 12-lead ECG.
- ◆ Obtain and review portable chest X-ray.
- ◆ Obtain problem-focused history.
- ◆ Obtain problem-focused physical examination.
- ◆ Consider causes (differential diagnoses).

Serious signs or symptoms?
Due to the bradycardia?

 Yes — **No**

Intervention sequence
- ◆ Atropine I.V. bolus
- ◆ Transcutaneous pacing if available
- ◆ Dopamine I.V. infusion
- ◆ Epinephrine I.V. infusion
- ◆ Isoproterenol I.V. infusion

Type II second-degree atrioventricular (AV) block or third-degree AV block?

 Yes — **No**

- ◆ Prepare for transvenous pacer.
- ◆ If symptoms develop, use transcutaneous pacemaker until transvenous pacer is placed.

Observe.

pacing for emergency treatment. Treatment of chronic, symptomatic sinus bradycardia requires insertion of a permanent pacemaker.

Sinus tachycardia
✦ Acceleration of firing of the SA node beyond its normal discharge rate
✦ Sinus rate > 100 beats/minute

SINUS TACHYCARDIA

Sinus tachycardia is an acceleration of the firing of the sinoatrial node beyond its normal discharge rate. Sinus tachycardia in an adult is characterized by a sinus rate of more than 100 beats/ minute. The rate rarely exceeds 180 beats/minute except during strenuous exercise; the maximum rate achievable with exercise decreases with age. (See *Recognizing sinus tachycardia* and *Bradycardia and tachycardia in children,* page 51.)

Causes
✦ Normal response to exercise, pain, stress, fever, or strong emotions
✦ Cardiac conditions (heart failure, cardiogenic shock, pericarditis)
✦ Other conditions (shock, anemia, respiratory distress, pulmonary embolism, sepsis, hyperthyroidism)
✦ Drugs (atropine, isoproterenol, aminophylline, dopamine, dobutamine, epinephrine, alcohol, caffeine, nicotine, amphetamines)

CAUSES

Sinus tachycardia may be a normal response to exercise, pain, stress, fever, or strong emotions, such as fear and anxiety. Other causes of sinus tachycardia include:
✦ certain cardiac conditions, such as heart failure, cardiogenic shock, and pericarditis
✦ other conditions, such as shock, anemia, respiratory distress, pulmonary embolism, sepsis, and hyperthyroidism where the increased heart rate serves as a compensatory mechanism
✦ drugs, such as atropine, isoproterenol, aminophylline, dopamine, dobutamine, epinephrine, alcohol, caffeine, nicotine, and amphetamines.

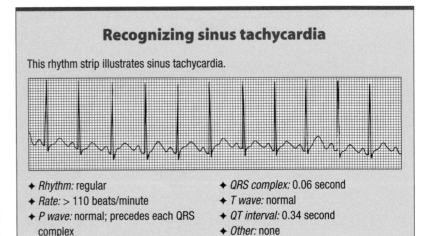

Recognizing sinus tachycardia

This rhythm strip illustrates sinus tachycardia.

✦ *Rhythm:* regular
✦ *Rate:* > 110 beats/minute
✦ *P wave:* normal; precedes each QRS complex
✦ *PR interval:* 0.14 second
✦ *QRS complex:* 0.06 second
✦ *T wave:* normal
✦ *QT interval:* 0.34 second
✦ *Other:* none

CLINICAL SIGNIFICANCE

The clinical significance of sinus tachycardia depends on the underlying cause. The arrhythmia may be the body's response to exercise or high emotional states and of no clinical significance. It may also occur with hypovolemia, hemorrhage, or pain. When the stimulus for the tachycardia is removed, the arrhythmia generally resolves spontaneously.

Although sinus tachycardia commonly occurs without serious adverse effects, persistent sinus tachycardia can also be serious, especially if it occurs in the setting of an acute myocardial infarction. Tachycardia can lower cardiac output by reducing ventricular filling time and stroke volume. Normally, ventricular volume reaches 120 to 130 ml during diastole. In tachycardia, decreased ventricular volume leads to decreased cardiac output with subsequent hypotension and decreased peripheral perfusion.

Tachycardia worsens myocardial ischemia by increasing the heart's demand for oxygen and reducing the duration of diastole, the period of greatest coronary blood flow. Sinus tachycardia occurs in about 30% of patients after an acute MI and is considered a poor prognostic sign because it may be associated with massive heart damage.

An increase in heart rate can also be detrimental for patients with obstructive types of heart conditions, such as aortic stenosis and hypertrophic cardiomyopathy. Persistent tachycardia may also signal impending heart failure or cardiogenic shock. Sinus tachycardia can also cause angina in patients with coronary artery disease.

ECG CHARACTERISTICS

+ *Rhythm*: Atrial and ventricular rhythms are regular.
+ *Rate:* Atrial and ventricular rates are greater than 100 beats/minute, usually between 100 and 160 beats/minute.
+ *P wave*: Normal size and configuration, but it may increase in amplitude. The P wave precedes each QRS complex, but as the heart rate increases, the P wave may be superimposed on the preceding T wave and difficult to identify.
+ *PR interval:* Within normal limits and constant.
+ *QRS complex:* Normal duration and configuration.
+ *T wave*: Normal size and configuration.
+ *QT interval:* Within normal limits, but commonly shortened.
+ *Other*: None.

SIGNS AND SYMPTOMS

The patient will have a peripheral pulse rate above 100 beats/minute, but with a regular rhythm. Usually, he'll be asymptomatic. However, if his cardiac

ECG characteristics

+ *Rhythm*—atrial and ventricular rhythms regular
+ *Rate*—atrial and ventricular rates > 100 beats/minute
+ *P wave*—normal size and configuration
+ *PR interval*—within normal limits and constant
+ *QRS complex*—normal duration and configuration
+ *QT interval*—within normal limits, but commonly shortened

Signs and symptoms

+ Peripheral pulse > 100 beats/minute; usually asymptomatic

Signs and symptoms
(continued)

If compensatory mechanisms fail

+ Hypotension
+ Syncope
+ Blurred vision
+ Chest pain, palpitations
+ Nervousness, anxiety
+ Crackles, S_3, jugular vein distention (if heart failure develops)

Interventions

+ Usually unnecessary, unless patient shows signs and symptoms of decreased cardiac output or hemodynamic instability
+ If symptomatic, identify and correct underlying cause

output falls and compensatory mechanisms fail, he may experience hypotension, syncope, and blurred vision. He may report chest pain and palpitations, commonly described as a pounding chest or a sensation of skipped heartbeats. He may also report a sense of nervousness or anxiety. If heart failure develops, he may exhibit crackles, an extra heart sound (S_3), and jugular vein distention.

INTERVENTIONS

Treatment usually isn't required unless the patient demonstrates signs and symptoms of decreased cardiac output or hemodynamic instability. The focus of treatment in the symptomatic patient with sinus tachycardia is to maintain adequate cardiac output and tissue perfusion and to identify and correct the underlying cause. For example, if the tachycardia is caused by hemorrhage, treatment includes stopping the bleeding and replacing blood and fluid losses.

If tachycardia leads to cardiac ischemia, treatment may include medications to slow the heart rate. The most commonly used drugs include beta-adrenergic blockers, such as propanolol and atenolol, and calcium channel blockers such as verapamil and diltiazem.

Check the patient's medication history. Over-the-counter sympathomimetic agents, which mimic the effects of the sympathetic nervous system, may contribute to the sinus tachycardia. Sympathomimetic agents may be contained in nose drops and cold formulas.

Also question the patient about the use of caffeine, nicotine, and alcohol, each of which can trigger tachycardia. Advise him to avoid these substances. Ask about the use of illicit drugs, such as cocaine and amphetamines, which can also cause tachycardia.

Here are other steps you should take for the patient with sinus tachycardia:

+ Because sinus tachycardia can lead to injury of the heart muscle, assess the patient for signs and symptoms of angina. Also assess for signs and symptoms of heart failure, including crackles, an S_3 heart sound, and jugular vein distention.
+ Monitor intake and output, along with daily weight.
+ Check the patient's level of consciousness to assess cerebral perfusion.
+ Provide the patient with a calm environment. Help to reduce fear and anxiety, which can aggravate the arrhythmia.
+ Teach about procedures and treatments. Include relaxation techniques in the information you provide.
+ Be aware that a sudden onset of sinus tachycardia after an MI may signal extension of the infarction. Prompt recognition is vital so treatment can be started.

✦ Keep in mind that tachycardia is frequently the initial sign of pulmonary embolism. Maintain a high index of suspicion, especially if your patient has predisposing risk factors for thrombotic emboli.

SINUS ARREST AND SINOATRIAL EXIT BLOCK

Although sinus arrest and sinoatrial (SA) or sinus exit block are two separate arrhythmias with different etiologies, they're discussed together because distinguishing the two can be difficult. In addition, there's no difference in their clinical significance and treatment.

In sinus arrest, the normal sinus rhythm is interrupted by an occasional, prolonged failure of the SA node to initiate an impulse. Therefore, sinus arrest is caused by episodes of failure in the automaticity or impulse formation of the SA node. The atria aren't stimulated, and an entire PQRST complex is missing from the ECG strip. Except for this missing complex, or pause, the ECG usually remains normal. (See *Recognizing sinus arrest.*)

In sinus exit block, the SA node discharges at regular intervals, but some impulses are delayed or blocked from reaching the atria, resulting in long sinus pauses. Blocks result from failure to conduct impulses, whereas sinus arrest results from failure to form impulses in the SA node. Both arrhythmias cause atrial activity to stop. In sinus arrest, the pause often ends with a junctional escape beat. In sinus exit block, the pause occurs for an indefinite period and ends with a sinus rhythm. (See *Recognizing sinoatrial exit block,* page 58.)

(See *Recognizing sinoatrial exit block,* page 58.)

(See *Recognizing sinus arrest.*)

Sinus arrest and SA exit block

✦ Sinus arrest — normal sinus rhythm interrupted by occasional, prolonged failure of SA node to initiate impulse
✦ SA exit block — SA node discharges at regular intervals, but some impulses delayed or blocked from reaching atria

---

Recognizing sinus arrest

This rhythm strip illustrates sinus arrest.

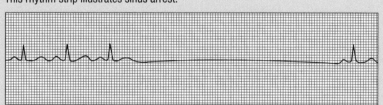

✦ *Rhythm:* regular, except for the missing PQRST complexes
✦ *Rate:* underlying rhythm, 75 beats/ minute
✦ *P wave:* normal; missing during pause
✦ *PR interval:* 0.20 second

✦ *QRS complex:* 0.08 second; missing during pause
✦ *T wave:* normal; missing during pause
✦ *QT interval:* 0.40 second; missing during pause
✦ *Other:* none

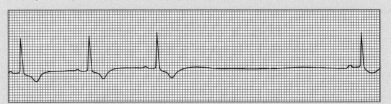

Recognizing sinoatrial exit block

This rhythm strip illustrates sinoatrial (SA) exit block.

- *Rhythm:* regular, except for pauses
- *Rate:* underlying rhythm, 60 beats/ minute before SA block; length or frequency of the pause may result in bradycardia
- *P wave:* periodically absent
- *PR interval:* 0.16 second
- *QRS complex:* 0.08 second; missing during pause
- *T wave:* normal; missing during pause
- *QT interval:* 0.40 second; missing during pause
- *Other:* entire PQRST complex missing; pause ends with sinus rhythm

Causes

- Acute infection
- SSS
- Sinus node diseases
- Increased vagal tone
- Digoxin, quinidine, procainamide, and salicylate toxicity
- Beta-adrenergic blockers (excessive doses)
- Cardiac disorders (CAD, acute myocarditis, cardiomyopathy, hypertensive heart disease, acute inferior wall MI)

CAUSES

Causes of sinus arrest and sinus exit block include:
- acute infection
- sick sinus syndrome
- sinus node diseases, such as fibrosis and idiopathic degeneration
- increased vagal tone, such as with Valsalva's maneuver, carotid sinus massage, and vomiting
- digoxin, quinidine, procainamide, and salicylate toxicity
- excessive doses of beta-adrenergic blockers, such as metoprolol and propranolol
- cardiac disorders, such as coronary artery disease (CAD), acute myocarditis, cardiomyopathy, hypertensive heart disease, and acute inferior wall myocardial infarction.

CLINICAL SIGNIFICANCE

The clinical significance of these two arrhythmias depends on the patient's symptoms. If the pauses are short and infrequent, the patient will most likely be asymptomatic and won't require treatment. He may have a normal sinus rhythm for days or weeks between episodes of sinus arrest or sinus exit block, and he may be totally unaware of the arrhythmia. Pauses of 2 to 3 seconds normally occur in healthy adults during sleep and occasionally in patients with increased vagal tone or hypersensitive carotid sinus disease.

If either of the arrhythmias is frequent or prolonged, however, the patient will most likely experience symptoms related to low cardiac output. The arrhythmias can produce syncope or near-syncopal episodes usually within 7 seconds of asystole.

During a prolonged pause, the patient may fall and injure himself. Other situations are potentially just as serious. For example, a symptom-producing arrhythmia that occurs while the patient is driving a car could result in a fatal accident. Extremely slow rates can also give rise to other arrhythmias.

ECG CHARACTERISTICS

Sinus arrest and SA exit block share these ECG characteristics:
+ *Rhythm:* Atrial and ventricular rhythms are usually regular except when sinus arrest or SA exit block occurs.
+ *Rate:* The underlying atrial and ventricular rates are usually within normal limits (60 to 100 beats/minute) before the arrest or SA exit block occurs. The length or frequency of the pause may result in bradycardia.
+ *P wave:* Periodically absent, with entire PQRST complex missing. However, when present, the P wave is normal in size and configuration and precedes each QRS complex.
+ *PR interval:* Within normal limits and constant when a P wave is present.
+ *QRS complex:* Normal duration and configuration, but absent during a pause.
+ *T wave:* Normal size and configuration, but absent during a pause.
+ *QT interval:* Usually within normal limits, but absent during a pause.

To differentiate between these two rhythms, compare the length of the pause with the underlying P-P or R-R interval. If the underlying rhythm is regular, determine if the underlying rhythm resumes on time following the pause. With sinus exit block, because the regularity of the SA node discharge is blocked, not interrupted, the underlying rhythm will resume on time following the pause. In addition, the length of the pause will be a multiple of the underlying P-P or R-R interval.

In sinus arrest, the timing of the SA node discharge is interrupted by the failure of the SA node to initiate an impulse. The result is that the underlying rhythm doesn't resume on time after the pause and the length of the pause is not a multiple of the previous R-R intervals.

SIGNS AND SYMPTOMS

You won't be able to detect a pulse or heart sounds when sinus arrest or sinus exit block occurs. Short pauses usually produce no symptoms. Recurrent or prolonged pauses may cause signs of decreased cardiac output, such as low blood pressure; altered mental status; cool, clammy skin; or syncope. The patient may also complain of dizziness or blurred vision.

ECG characteristics
+ *Rhythm*—atrial and ventricular rhythms usually regular except when sinus arrest or SA exit block occurs
+ *Rate*—underlying atrial and ventricular rates usually within normal limits before arrest or SA exit block occurs
+ *P wave*—periodically absent, with entire PQRST complex missing
+ *PR interval*—within normal limits and constant (when P wave is present)
+ *QRS complex*—normal duration and configuration (absent during pause)

Signs and symptoms
Short pauses
+ No symptoms

Recurrent or prolonged pauses
+ Low blood pressure
+ Altered mental status
+ Cool, clammy skin
+ Syncope
+ Dizziness, blurred vision

Interventions

+ Unnecessary for asymptomatic patient
+ If symptomatic, focus on cause of sinus arrest or sinus exit block

INTERVENTIONS

An asymptomatic patient needs no treatment. Symptomatic patients are treated following the guidelines for patients with symptom-producing bradycardia. (See *Bradycardia algorithm*, page 53.) Treatment will also focus on the cause of the sinus arrest or sinus exit block. This may involve discontinuation of medications that contribute to SA node discharge or conduction, such as digoxin, beta-adrenergic blockers, and calcium channel blockers.

Examine the circumstances under which the pauses occur. Both SA arrest and SA exit block may be insignificant if detected while the patient is sleeping. If the pauses are recurrent, assess the patient for evidence of decreased cardiac output, such as altered mental status, low blood pressure, and cool, clammy skin.

Ask him whether he's dizzy or light-headed or has blurred vision. Does he feel as if he has passed out? If so, he may be experiencing syncope from a prolonged sinus arrest or sinus exit block.

Document the patient's vital signs and how he feels during pauses as well as the activities he was involved in at the time. Activities that increase vagal stimulation, such as Valsalva's maneuver or vomiting, increase the likelihood of sinus pauses.

Assess for a progression of the arrhythmia. Notify the physician immediately if the patient becomes unstable. If appropriate, be alert for signs of digoxin, quinidine, or procainamide toxicity. Obtain a serum digoxin level and a serum electrolyte level.

Sick sinus syndrome

+ Disturbances in way impulses are generated or in ability to conduct impulses to atria
+ Often appears as bradycardia, with sinus arrest and SA block mixed with brief periods of rapid atrial fibrillation
+ Patients more prone to paroxysms of other atrial tachyarrhythmias

SICK SINUS SYNDROME

Also known as *sinoatrial (SA) syndrome, sinus nodal dysfunction,* and *Stokes-Adams syndrome,* sick sinus syndrome (SSS) refers to a wide spectrum of SA node arrhythmias. This syndrome is caused by disturbances in the way impulses are generated or in the ability to conduct impulses to the atria. These disturbances may be either intrinsic or mediated by the autonomic nervous system (ANS).

SSS usually shows up as bradycardia, with episodes of sinus arrest and SA block interspersed with sudden, brief periods of rapid atrial fibrillation. Patients are also prone to paroxysms of other atrial tachyarrhythmias, such as atrial flutter and ectopic atrial tachycardia, a condition sometimes referred to as *bradycardia-tachycardia* (or *"brady-tachy"*) *syndrome.*

Most patients with SSS are over age 60, but anyone can develop the arrhythmia. It's rare in children except after open-heart surgery that results in SA node damage. The arrhythmia affects men and women equally. The onset is progressive, insidious, and chronic. (See *Recognizing sick sinus syndrome.*)

Recognizing sick sinus syndrome

This rhythm strip illustrates sick sinus syndrome.

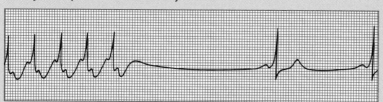

- ✦ *Rhythm:* irregular
- ✦ *Rate:* atrial and ventricular rates fast (150 beats/minute) or slow (43 beats/minute) or alternate between fast and slow; interrupted by a long sinus pause
- ✦ *P wave:* varies with prevailing rhythm
- ✦ *PR interval:* varies with rhythm
- ✦ *QRS complex:* 0.10 second; may vary with rhythm
- ✦ *T wave:* configuration varies
- ✦ *QT interval:* varies with rhythm changes
- ✦ *Other:* sinus pause due to nonfiring sinus node

CAUSES

SSS results either from a dysfunction of the sinus node's automaticity or from abnormal conduction or blockages of impulses coming out of the nodal region. These conditions, in turn, stem from a degeneration of the area's ANS and partial destruction of the sinus node, as may occur with an interrupted blood supply after an inferior wall myocardial infarction.

In addition, certain conditions can affect the atrial wall surrounding the SA node and cause exit blocks. Conditions that cause inflammation or degeneration of atrial tissue can also lead to SSS. In many patients, though, the exact cause is never identified.

Causes of SSS include:

✦ conditions leading to fibrosis of the SA node, such as increased age, atherosclerotic heart disease, hypertension, and cardiomyopathy

✦ trauma to the SA node caused by open heart surgery (especially valvular surgery), pericarditis, or rheumatic heart disease

✦ autonomic disturbances affecting autonomic innervation, such as hypervagotonia or degeneration of the autonomic system

✦ cardioactive medications, such as digoxin, beta-adrenergic antagonists, and calcium channel blockers.

Causes

✦ Dysfunction of SA node's automaticity or abnormal conduction or blockages of impulses out of region
✦ Conditions leading to fibrosis of SA node
✦ Trauma to SA node caused by open heart surgery, pericarditis, or rheumatic heart disease
✦ Autonomic disturbances affecting autonomic innervation
✦ Digoxin, beta-adrenergic antagonists, and calcium channel blockers

CLINICAL SIGNIFICANCE

The significance of SSS depends on the patient's age, the presence of other diseases, and the type and duration of the specific arrhythmias that occur. If atrial fibrillation is involved, the prognosis is worse, most likely because of the risk of thromboembolic complications.

If prolonged pauses are involved with SSS, syncope may occur. The length of a pause needed to cause syncope varies with the patient's age, posture at the time, and cerebrovascular status. Any pause that lasts 2 to 3 seconds or more should be considered significant.

A significant part of the diagnosis is whether the patient experiences symptoms while the disturbance occurs. Because the syndrome is progressive and chronic, a symptomatic patient will need lifelong treatment. In addition, thromboembolism may develop as a complication of SSS, possibly resulting in stroke or peripheral embolization.

ECG characteristics

+ *Rhythm*—atrial and ventricular rhythms irregular due to sinus pauses and abrupt rate changes
+ *Rate*—atrial and ventricular rates fast or slow or alternate between the two
+ *P wave*—varies with prevailing rhythm
+ *PR interval*—usually within normal limits; varies with rhythm changes
+ *QRS complex*—usually within normal limits; varies with rhythm changes

ECG CHARACTERISTICS

SSS encompasses several potential rhythm disturbances that may be intermittent or chronic. SSS may include one, or a combination, of these rhythm disturbances:
+ sinus bradycardia
+ SA block
+ sinus arrest
+ sinus bradycardia alternating with sinus tachycardia
+ episodes of atrial tachyarrhythmias, such as atrial fibrillation and atrial flutter
+ failure of the sinus node to increase heart rate with exercise.

SSS displays these ECG characteristics:
+ *Rhythm:* atrial and ventricular rhythms irregular because of sinus pauses and abrupt rate changes
+ *Rate:* atrial and ventricular rates are fast or slow or alternate between fast and slow; and interrupted by a long sinus pause
+ *P wave:* varies with the prevailing rhythm; may be normal size and configuration or may be absent; when present, a P wave usually precedes each QRS complex
+ *PR interval:* usually within normal limits; varies with change in rhythm
+ *QRS complex:* duration usually within normal limits; may vary with changes in rhythm; usually normal configuration
+ *T wave:* usually normal size and configuration
+ *QT interval:* usually within normal limits; varies with rhythm changes
+ *Other:* usually more than one arrhythmia on a 6-second strip.

Check mental status

Because the older adult with sick sinus syndrome may have mental status changes, be sure to perform a thorough assessment to rule out such disorders as stroke, delirium, or dementia.

SIGNS AND SYMPTOMS

The patient's pulse rate may be fast, slow, or normal, and the rhythm may be regular or irregular. You can usually detect an irregularity on the monitor or when palpating the pulse, which may feel inappropriately slow, then rapid.

If you monitor the patient's heart rate during exercise or exertion, you may observe an inappropriate response to exercise, such as a failure of the heart rate to increase. You may also detect episodes of brady-tachy syndrome, atrial flutter, atrial fibrillation, SA block, or sinus arrest on the monitor.

Other assessment findings depend on the patient's condition. For example, he may have crackles in the lungs, S_3, or a dilated and displaced left ventricular apical impulse if he has underlying cardiomyopathy. The patient may also show signs and symptoms of decreased cardiac output, such as fatigue, hypotension, blurred vision, and syncope, a common experience with this arrhythmia. Syncopal episodes, when related to SSS, are referred to as *Stokes-Adams attacks*.

When caring for a patient with SSS, be alert for signs and symptoms of thromboembolism, especially if the patient has atrial fibrillation. Blood clots or thrombi forming in the heart can dislodge and travel through the bloodstream, resulting in decreased blood supply to the lungs, heart, brain, kidneys, intestines, or other organs. Assess the patient for neurologic changes (such as confusion), vision disturbances, weakness, chest pain, dyspnea, tachypnea, tachycardia, and acute onset of pain. Early recognition allows for prompt treatment. (See *Check mental status*.)

INTERVENTIONS

As with other sinus node arrhythmias, no treatment is generally necessary if the patient is asymptomatic. If the patient is symptomatic, however, treatment aims to alleviate signs and symptoms and correct the underlying cause of the arrhythmia.

Signs and symptoms
+ Pulse rate fast, slow, or normal; rhythm regular or irregular
+ Crackles in lungs, S_3, or dilated and displaced left ventricular apical impulse (with underlying cardiomyopathy
+ Fatigue, hypotension, blurred vision, and syncope (with decreased cardiac output)
+ Thromboembolism (with atrial fibrillation)

Interventions
+ Unnecessary in asymptomatic patients
+ If symptomatic, focus on correcting underlying cause

Atropine or epinephrine may be given initially for symptom-producing bradycardia. (See *Bradycardia algorithm,* page 53.) A temporary pacemaker may be required until the underlying disorder resolves. Tachyarrhythmias may be treated with antiarrhythmic medications, such as metoprolol and digoxin. Unfortunately, medications used to suppress tachyarrhythmias may worsen underlying SA node disease and bradyarrhythmias.

The patient may need anticoagulants if he develops sudden bursts, or paroxysms, of atrial fibrillation. The anticoagulants help prevent thromboembolism and stroke, a complication of the condition.

When caring for a patient with SSS, monitor and document all arrhythmias as well as signs or symptoms experienced. Note changes in heart rate and rhythm related to changes in the patient's level of activity.

Watch the patient carefully after starting beta-adrenergic blockers, calcium channel blockers, or other antiarrhythmic medications. If treatment includes anticoagulant therapy and pacemaker insertion, make sure the patient and his family receive appropriate instruction.

Atrial arrhythmias

Atrial arrhythmias, the most common cardiac rhythm disturbances, result from impulses originating in the atrial tissue in areas outside the sinoatrial (SA) node. These arrhythmias can affect ventricular filling time and diminish atrial kick. The term *atrial kick* refers to the complete filling of the ventricles during atrial systole and normally contributes about 25% to ventricular end-diastolic volume.

Atrial arrhythmias are thought to result from three mechanisms: altered automaticity, reentry, and afterdepolarization.

✦ *Altered automaticity.* The term automaticity refers to the ability of cardiac cells to initiate electrical impulses spontaneously. An increase in the automaticity of the atrial fibers can trigger abnormal impulses. Causes of increased automaticity include extracellular factors, such as hypoxia, hypocalcemia, and digoxin toxicity as well as conditions in which the function of the heart's normal pacemaker, the SA node, is diminished. For example, increased vagal tone or hypokalemia can increase the refractory period of the SA node and allow atrial fibers to initiate impulses.

✦ *Reentry.* In reentry, an impulse is delayed along a slow conduction pathway. Despite the delay, the impulse remains active enough to produce another impulse during myocardial repolarization. Reentry may occur with coronary artery disease, cardiomyopathy, or myocardial infarction.

✦ *Afterdepolarization.* Afterdepolarization can occur as a result of cell injury, digoxin toxicity, and other conditions. An injured cell sometimes only partially repolarizes. Partial repolarization can lead to repetitive ectopic firing called *triggered activity.* The depolarization produced by triggered activity, known as *afterdepolarization,* can lead to atrial or ventricular tachycardia.

Atrial arrhythmias

✦ Impulses originate in atrial tissue in areas outside SA node
✦ Impact ventricular filling time and diminish atrial kick

Three mechanisms

✦ *Altered automaticity*—increase in automaticity of atrial fibers trigger abnormal impulses
✦ *Reentry*—impulse delayed along slow conduction pathway
✦ *Afterdepolarization*—can occur as result of cell injury or digoxin toxicity

This chapter will help you identify atrial arrhythmias, including premature atrial contractions, atrial tachycardia, atrial flutter, atrial fibrillation, Ashman's phenomenon, and wandering pacemaker. The chapter reviews causes, clinical significance, electrocardiogram (ECG) characteristics, and signs and symptoms of each arrhythmia as well as interventions directed at treating the patient experiencing these arrhythmias.

Premature atrial contractions

+ Originate in atria, outside SA node
+ Arise from single ectopic focus or multiple atrial foci, superseding SA node as pacemaker for one or more beats
+ When conducted, ventricular conduction usually normal; when blocked, not followed by QRS complex

PREMATURE ATRIAL CONTRACTIONS

Premature atrial contractions (PACs) originate in the atria, outside the sinoatrial (SA) node. They arise from either a single ectopic focus or from multiple atrial foci that supersede the SA node as pacemaker for one or more beats. PACs are generally caused by enhanced automaticity in the atrial tissue. (See *Recognizing premature atrial contractions*.)

PACs may be conducted or nonconducted (blocked) through the atrioventricular (AV) node and the rest of the heart, depending on the status of the AV and intraventricular conduction system. If the atrial ectopic pacemaker discharges too soon after the preceding QRS complex, the AV junction or bundle branches may still be refractory from conducting the previous electrical impulse. If they're still refractory, they may not be sufficiently repolarized to conduct the premature electrical impulse into the ventricles normally.

When a PAC is conducted, ventricular conduction is usually normal. Nonconducted, or blocked, PACs aren't followed by a QRS complex. At times, it may be difficult to distinguish nonconducted PACs from SA block. (See *Distinguishing nonconducted premature atrial contractions from sinoatrial block*.)

Recognizing premature atrial contractions

This rhythm strip illustrates sinus rhythm with premature atrial contractions (PACs).

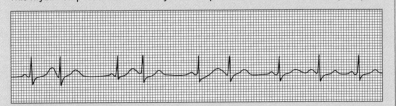

+ *Rhythm:* irregular
+ *Rate:* 90 beats/minute
+ *P wave:* premature and abnormally shaped with PACs
+ *PR interval:* 0.20 second for the underlying rhythm; unmeasureable for the PAC
+ *QRS complex:* 0.08 second
+ *T wave:* abnormal with embedded P waves of PACs
+ *QT interval:* 0.32 second
+ *Other:* noncompensatory pause

Distinguishing nonconducted premature atrial contractions from sinoatrial block

To differentiate nonconducted premature atrial contractions (PACs) from sinoatrial (SA) block, check the following:

✦ Whenever you see a pause in a rhythm, look carefully for a nonconducted P wave, which may occur before, during, or just after the T wave preceding the pause.

✦ Compare T waves that precede a pause with the other T waves in the rhythm strip, and look for a distortion of the slope of the T wave or a difference in its height or shape. These are clues showing you where the nonconducted P wave may be hidden.

✦ If you find a P wave in the pause, check to see whether it's premature or if it occurs earlier than subsequent sinus P waves. If it's premature (see shaded area below, top), you can be certain it's a nonconducted PAC.

✦ If there's no P wave in the pause or T wave (see shaded area below, bottom), the rhythm is SA block.

NONCONDUCTED PAC

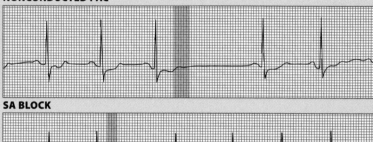

SA BLOCK

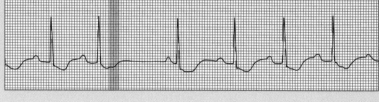

Causes

Alcohol, cigarettes, anxiety, fatigue, fever, and infectious diseases can trigger PACs, which commonly occur in a normal heart. Patients who eliminate or control those factors can usually correct the arrhythmia.

PACs may be associated with hyperthyroidism, coronary or valvular heart disease, acute respiratory failure, hypoxia, chronic pulmonary disease, digoxin toxicity, and certain electrolyte imbalances. PACs may also be caused by drugs that prolong the absolute refractory period of the SA node, including quinidine and procainamide.

Causes

✦ Alcohol
✦ Cigarettes
✦ Anxiety
✦ Fatigue
✦ Fever
✦ Infectious diseases

CLINICAL SIGNIFICANCE

PACs are rarely dangerous in patients free of heart disease. They often cause no symptoms and can go unrecognized for years. Patients may perceive PACs as normal palpitations or skipped beats.

However, in patients with heart disease, PACs may lead to more serious arrhythmias, such as atrial fibrillation or atrial flutter. In a patient with acute myocardial infarction, PACs can serve as an early sign of heart failure or electrolyte imbalance. PACs can also result from endogenous catecholamine release during episodes of pain or anxiety.

ECG characteristics

+ *Rhythm*—atrial and ventricular rhythms irregular
+ *Rate*—atrial and ventricular rates vary with underlying rhythm
+ *P wave*—premature with abnormal configuration (when compared with sinus P wave)
+ *QRS complex*—duration and configuration usually normal
+ *Other*—three or more PACs in a row (atrial tachycardia)

ECG CHARACTERISTICS

+ *Rhythm:* Atrial and ventricular rhythms are irregular as a result of PACs, but the underlying rhythm may be regular.
+ *Rate*: Atrial and ventricular rates vary with the underlying rhythm.
+ *P wave:* The hallmark characteristic of a PAC is a premature P wave with an abnormal configuration, when compared with a sinus P wave. Varying configurations of the P wave indicate more than one ectopic site. PACs may be hidden in the preceding T wave.
+ *PR interval*: Usually within normal limits but may be either shortened or slightly prolonged for the ectopic beat, depending on the origin of the ectopic focus.
+ *QRS complex:* Duration and configuration are usually normal when the PAC is conducted. If no QRS complex follows the PAC, the beat is called a *nonconducted PAC*.
+ *T wave:* Usually normal; however, if the P wave is hidden in the T wave, the T wave may appear distorted.
+ *QT interval:* Usually within normal limits.
+ *Other:* PACs may occur as a single beat, in a bigeminal (every other beat is premature), trigeminal (every third beat), or quadrigeminal (every fourth beat) pattern, or in couplets (pairs). Three or more PACs in a row is called *atrial tachycardia.*

PACs are commonly followed by a pause as the SA node resets. The PAC depolarizes the SA node early, causing it to reset itself and disrupting the normal cycle. The next sinus beat occurs sooner than it normally would, causing a P-P interval between normal beats interrupted by a PAC to be shorter than three consecutive sinus beats, an occurrence referred to as *noncompensatory.*

Signs and symptoms

+ Irregular peripheral or apical pulse rhythm

SIGNS AND SYMPTOMS

The patient may have an irregular peripheral or apical pulse rhythm when the PACs occur. Otherwise, the pulse rhythm and rate will reflect the underlying rhythm. Patients may complain of palpitations, skipped beats, or a fluttering sensation. In a patient with heart disease, signs and symptoms of decreased cardiac output, such as hypotension and syncope, may occur.

INTERVENTIONS

Most asymptomatic patients don't need treatment. If the patient is symptomatic, however, treatment may focus on eliminating the cause, such as caffeine and alcohol. People with frequent PACs may be treated with drugs that prolong the refractory period of the atria. Those drugs include beta-adrenergic blockers and calcium channel blockers.

When caring for a patient with PACs, assess him to help determine factors that trigger ectopic beats. Tailor patient teaching to help the patient correct or avoid underlying causes. For example, the patient might need to avoid caffeine or learn stress reduction techniques to lessen anxiety.

If the patient has ischemic or valvular heart disease, monitor for signs and symptoms of heart failure, electrolyte imbalance, and more severe atrial arrhythmias.

ATRIAL TACHYCARDIA

Atrial tachycardia is a supraventricular tachycardia, which means that the impulses driving the rapid rhythm originate above the ventricles. Atrial tachycardia has an atrial rate from 150 to 250 beats/minute. The rapid rate shortens diastole, resulting in a loss of atrial kick, reduced cardiac output, reduced coronary perfusion, and the potential for myocardial ischemia. (See *Recognizing atrial tachycardia*.)

Recognizing atrial tachycardia

This rhythm strip illustrates atrial tachycardia.

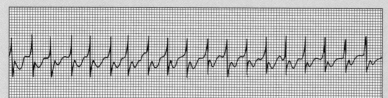

+ *Rhythm:* regular
+ *Rate:* 210 beats/minute
+ *P wave:* hidden in the preceding T wave
+ *PR interval:* not visible
+ *QRS complex:* 0.10 second
+ *T wave:* inverted
+ *QT interval:* 0.20 second
+ *Other:* T-wave changes (inversion may indicate ischemia)

Signs and symptoms
(continued)
+ Palpitations, skipped beats, fluttering sensation, or hypotension

Interventions
+ Unnecessary for asymptomatic patients; if symptomatic, focus on eliminating cause

Atrial tachycardia
+ Impulses driving rapid rhythm originate above ventricles (supraventricular tachycardia)

Atrial tachycardia
(continued)

Three forms
+ Atrial tachycardia with block
+ MAT or chaotic atrial rhythm
+ PAT

Causes
+ Caffeine or other stimulants (excessive)
+ Electrolyte imbalance, hypoxia, or physical or psychological stress
+ Cardiac disorders (valvular heart disease)

ECG characteristics
+ *Rhythm*—atrial rhythm usually regular; ventricular rhythm varies, depending on AV conduction ratio
+ *Rate*—between 150 and 250 beats/minute
+ *P wave*—possibly aberrant or hidden in preceding T wave

Three forms of atrial tachycardia are discussed here: atrial tachycardia with block, multifocal atrial tachycardia (MAT, or chaotic atrial rhythm), and paroxysmal atrial tachycardia (PAT). In MAT, the tachycardia originates from multiple foci. PAT is generally a transient event in which the tachycardia appears and disappears suddenly.

CAUSES

Atrial tachycardia can occur in patients with a normal heart. In those cases, it's commonly related to excessive use of caffeine or other stimulants, marijuana use, electrolyte imbalance, hypoxia, or physical or psychological stress. Typically, however, atrial tachycardia is associated with primary or secondary cardiac disorders, including myocardial infarction (MI), cardiomyopathy, congenital anomalies, Wolff-Parkinson-White (WPW) syndrome, and valvular heart disease.

This rhythm may be a component of sick sinus syndrome. Other problems resulting in atrial tachycardia include cor pulmonale, hyperthyroidism, systemic hypertension, and digoxin toxicity, the most common cause of atrial tachycardia.

CLINICAL SIGNIFICANCE

In a healthy person, nonsustained atrial tachycardia is usually benign. However, this rhythm may be a forerunner of more serious ventricular arrhythmias, especially if it occurs in a patient with underlying heart disease.

The increased ventricular rate that occurs in atrial tachycardia results in decreased ventricular filling time, increased myocardial oxygen consumption, and decreased oxygen supply to the myocardium. Heart failure, myocardial ischemia, and MI can result.

ECG CHARACTERISTICS

+ *Rhythm:* The atrial rhythm is usually regular. The ventricular rhythm is regular or irregular, depending on the atrioventricular (AV) conduction ratio and the type of atrial tachycardia. (See *Identifying types of atrial tachycardia.*)
+ *Rate:* The atrial rate is characterized by three or more consecutive ectopic atrial beats occurring at a rate between 150 and 250 beats/minute. The rate rarely exceeds 250 beats/minute. The ventricular rate depends on the AV conduction ratio.
+ *P wave:* The P wave may be aberrant (deviating from normal appearance) or hidden in the preceding T wave. If visible, it's usually upright and precedes each QRS complex.
+ *PR interval:* The PR interval may be unmeasurable if the P wave can't be distinguished from the preceding T wave.

Identifying types of atrial tachycardia

Characteristics of atrial tachycardia with block:

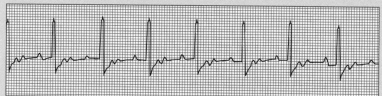

- ✦ *Rhythm:* atrial — regular; ventricular — regular if block is constant; irregular if block is variable
- ✦ *Rate:* atrial — 140 to 250 beats/minute and a multiple of ventricular rate; ventricular — varies with block
- ✦ *P wave:* slightly abnormal
- ✦ *PR interval:* can vary but is usually constant for conducted P waves
- ✦ *QRS complex:* usually normal
- ✦ *T wave:* usually indistinguishable
- ✦ *QT interval:* may be indiscernible
- ✦ *Other:* more than one P wave for each QRS

Characteristics of multifocal atrial tachycardia:

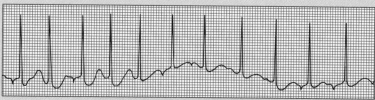

- ✦ *Rhythm:* both irregular
- ✦ *Rate:* atrial — 100 to 250 beats/minute; ventricular — 100 to 250 beats/minute
- ✦ *P wave:* configuration varies; usually at least three different P-wave shapes must appear
- ✦ *PR interval:* varies
- ✦ *QRS complex:* usually normal, may become aberrant if arrhythmia persists
- ✦ *T wave:* usually distorted
- ✦ *QT interval:* may be indiscernible
- ✦ *Other:* none

Characteristics of paroxysmal atrial tachycardia:

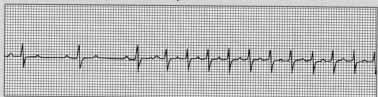

- ✦ *Rhythm:* atrial and ventricular rhythms may be regular or irregular and start and stop abruptly
- ✦ *Rate:* 140 to 250 beats/minute
- ✦ *P wave:* may be retrograde; may not be visible or may be difficult to distinguish from the preceding T wave
- ✦ *PR interval:* may be unmeasurable if the P wave can't be distinguished from the preceding T wave
- ✦ *QRS complex:* can be aberrantly conducted
- ✦ *T wave:* usually indistinguishable
- ✦ *QT interval:* may be indistinguishable
- ✦ *Other:* sudden onset, typically initiated by a premature atrial contraction

ECG characteristics
(continued)
+ *QRS complex*—duration and configuration usually normal

Signs and symptoms
+ Palpitations
+ Hypotension and syncope (decreased cardiac output)

Interventions
+ Depends on type of tachycardia and severity of symptoms
+ Valsalva maneuver or carotid sinus massage (for PAT)
+ Drugs (adenosine, amiodarone, beta-adrenergic blockers, calcium channel blockers)
+ Synchronized electrical cardioversion (if other treatments fail or if patient is clinically unstable)
+ Atrial overdrive pacing
+ Catheter ablation, if arrhythmia is associated with WPW syndrome (for recurrent PAT)

+ *QRS complex:* Duration and configuration are usually normal, unless the impulses are being conducted abnormally through the ventricles.
+ *T wave:* Usually distinguishable but may be distorted by the P wave; may be inverted if ischemia is present.
+ *QT interval:* Usually within normal limits but may be shorter because of the rapid rate.
+ *Other:* Sometimes it may be difficult to distinguish atrial tachycardia with block from sinus arrhythmia with U waves. (See *Distinguishing atrial tachycardia with block from sinus arrhythmia with U waves.*)

SIGNS AND SYMPTOMS

The patient with atrial tachycardia will have a rapid apical and peripheral pulse rate. The rhythm may be regular or irregular, depending on the type of atrial tachycardia. A patient with PAT may complain that his heart suddenly starts to beat faster or that he suddenly feels palpitations. Persistent tachycardia and rapid ventricular rate cause decreased cardiac output, resulting in hypotension and syncope.

INTERVENTIONS

Treatment depends on the type of tachycardia and the severity of the patient's symptoms. (See *Tachycardia algorithm,* pages 74 and 75.) Because one of the most common causes of atrial tachycardia is digoxin toxicity, assess the patient for signs and symptoms of digoxin toxicity and monitor digoxin blood levels.

The Valsalva maneuver or carotid sinus massage may be used to treat PAT. (See *Understanding carotid sinus massage,* page 76.) These maneuvers increase the parasympathetic tone, which results in a slowing of the heart rate. They also allow the sinoatrial (SA) node to resume function as the primary pacemaker.

If vagal maneuvers are used, make sure resuscitative equipment is readily available. (See *Avoid carotid massage in elderly patients,* page 76.) Keep in mind that vagal stimulation can result in bradycardia, ventricular arrhythmias, and asystole. (See *Narrow-complex tachycardia algorithm,* page 77.)

Drug therapy (pharmacologic cardioversion) may be used to increase the degree of AV block and decrease ventricular response rate. Appropriate drugs include adenosine, amiodarone, beta-adrenergic blockers, calcium channel blockers, and digoxin. When other treatments fail, or if the patient is clinically unstable, synchronized electrical cardioversion may be used.

Atrial overdrive pacing (also called *rapid atrial pacing* or *overdrive suppression*) may also be used to stop the arrhythmia. This technique involves suppression of spontaneous depolarization of the ectopic pacemaker by a series of paced electrical impulses at a rate slightly higher than the intrinsic ec-

Distinguishing atrial tachycardia with block from sinus arrhythmia with U waves

Atrial tachycardia with block may appear strikingly similar to sinus arrhythmia with U waves. Always check "normal" rhythm strips carefully to make sure you haven't overlooked or misinterpreted something abnormal. Here's how to tell the difference between the two rhythms.

ATRIAL TACHYCARDIA WITH BLOCK

✦ Examine the T wave and the interval from the T wave to the next P wave for evidence of extra P waves (see shaded areas below). If you find extra P waves, map them to determine whether they occur at regular intervals with the "normal" P waves.

✦ In atrial tachycardia with block, the P-P intervals are constant.

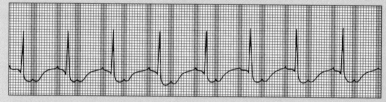

SINUS ARRHYTHMIA WITH U WAVES

✦ It's possible to mistake a U wave (see shaded areas below) for an extra P wave. The key is to determine if all of the waves occur at regular intervals. In sinus arrhythmia with U waves, the interval from a U wave to a P wave and a P wave to a U wave won't be constant.

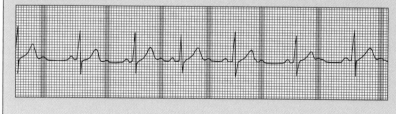

topic atrial rate. The pacemaker cells are depolarized prematurely and, following termination of the paced electrical impulses, the SA node resumes its normal role as the pacemaker.

If the arrhythmia is associated with WPW syndrome, catheter ablation (permanent damage of the area causing the arrhythmia) may be used to control recurrent episodes of PAT. Because MAT commonly occurs in patients with chronic pulmonary disease, the rhythm may not respond to treatment.

(*Text continues on page 78.*)

Tachycardia algorithm

The algorithm for tachycardia is complex. Remember to base your actions on the type of tachycardia the patient is experiencing and how he's tolerating the rhythm.

Evaluate patient.
✦ Is patient stable or unstable?
✦ Are there serious signs or symptoms?
✦ Are signs and symptoms due to tachycardia?

STABLE

No serious signs or symptoms
✦ Initial assessment identifies one of four types of tachycardia.

Atrial fibrillation or atrial flutter

Narrow-complex tachycardias

Focus evaluation on four clinical features.
✦ Patient clinically unstable?
✦ Cardiac function impaired?
✦ Wolff-Parkinson-White syndrome present?
✦ Duration < 48 or > 48 hours?

Attempt to establish a specific diagnosis.
✦ 12-lead ECG
✦ Clinical information
✦ Vagal maneuvers
✦ Adenosine

Focus treatment on four elements.
✦ Treat unstable patients urgently.
✦ Control the rate.
✦ Convert the rhythm.
✦ Provide anticoagulation.

Possible diagnoses
✦ Ectopic atrial tachycardia
✦ Multifocal atrial tachycardia
✦ Paroxysmal supraventricular tachycardia (PSVT)

Follow treatment for atrial fibrillation/atrial flutter.

See narrow-complex tachycardia algorithm.

UNSTABLE

Serious signs or symptoms
+ Signs and symptoms are the result of rapid heart rate
  (> 150 beats/minute); prepare for immediate cardioversion.

Stable wide-complex tachycardia: unknown type	**See stable monomorphic or polymorphic ventricular tachycardia (VT) algorithm**

Attempt to establish a specific diagnosis.
+ 12-lead ECG
+ Esophageal lead
+ Clinical information

Confirmed PSVT	**Wide-complex tachycardia of unknown type**	**Confirmed stable VT**

Preserved cardiac function	**Impaired heart (ejection fraction < 40%), clinical heart failure**
Cardioversion, procainamide, or amiodarone	**Cardioversion or amiodarone**

Understanding carotid sinus massage

Carotid sinus massage may be used to interrupt paroxysmal atrial tachycardia. Massaging the carotid sinus stimulates the vagus nerve, which inhibits firing of the sinoatrial (SA) node and slows atrioventricular (AV) node conduction. As a result, the SA node can resume its function as primary pacemaker.

Carotid sinus massage involves a firm massage that lasts no longer than 5 to 10 seconds. The patient's head is turned to the left to massage the right carotid sinus, as shown below. Remember that simultaneous, bilateral massage should never be attempted.

Carotid sinus massage is contraindicated in patients with carotid bruits. Risks of the procedure include decreased heart rate, syncope, sinus arrest, increased degree of AV block, cerebral emboli, stroke, and asystole.

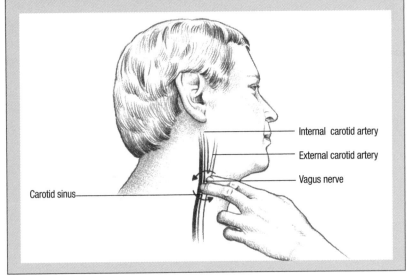

Internal carotid artery

External carotid artery

Vagus nerve

Carotid sinus

AGE CHANGE

Avoid carotid sinus massage in elderly patients

Older adults may have undiagnosed carotid atherosclerosis and carotid bruits may be absent, even with significant disease. As a result, cardiac sinus massage shouldn't be performed in late-middle-age and older patients.

Narrow-complex tachycardia algorithm

Types of narrow-complex tachycardia include junctional tachycardia, paroxysmal supraventricular tachycardia (PSVT), and multifocal atrial tachycardia (MAT). Treatment for each type of rhythm depends on how well the patient tolerates the rhythm.

Narrow-complex tachycardia, stable

Attempt therapeutic diagnostic maneuver.
- Vagal stimulation
- Adenosine

Junctional tachycardia

Preserved	Ejection fraction < 40%, heart failure
- Amiodarone - Beta-adrenergic blocker - Calcium channel blocker - No cardioversion!	- Amiodarone - No cardioversion!

PSVT

Preserved	Ejection fraction < 40%, heart failure
Treatments, in order of priority - Calcium channel blocker - Beta-adrenergic blocker - Digoxin - Cardioversion - Consider procainamide, amiodarone, sotalol	**Treatments, in order of priority** - No cardioversion! - Digoxin - Amiodarone - Diltiazem

Ectopic or MAT

Preserved	Ejection fraction < 40%, heart failure
- Calcium channel blocker - Beta-adrenergic blocker - Amiodarone - No cardioversion!	- Amiodarone - Diltiazem - No cardioversion!

When caring for a patient with atrial tachycardia, carefully monitor the patient's rhythm strips. Doing so may provide information about the cause of atrial tachycardia, which in turn can facilitate treatment. Monitor the patient for chest pain, indications of decreased cardiac output, and signs and symptoms of heart failure or myocardial ischemia.

ATRIAL FLUTTER

Atrial flutter
+ Rapid atrial rate of 250 to 400 beats/minute

Atrial flutter, a supraventricular tachycardia, is characterized by a rapid atrial rate of 250 to 400 beats/minute, although it's generally around 300 beats/minute. Originating in a single atrial focus, this rhythm results from circus reentry and possibly increased automaticity.

On an ECG, the P waves lose their normal appearance due to the rapid atrial rate. The waves blend together in a sawtooth configuration called *flutter waves,* or *F waves.* These waves are the hallmark of atrial flutter. (See *Recognizing atrial flutter.*)

CAUSES

Causes
+ Mitral or tricuspid valvular disease
+ Hyperthyroidism
+ Pericardial disease
+ Digoxin toxicity
+ Primary myocardial disease
+ Cardiac surgery
+ Acute MI
+ Chronic pulmonary disease
+ Systemic arterial hypoxia

Atrial flutter may be caused by conditions that enlarge atrial tissue and elevate atrial pressures. The arrhythmia is commonly found in patients with mitral or tricuspid valvular disease, hyperthyroidism, pericardial disease, digoxin toxicity, or primary myocardial disease. The rhythm is sometimes

---

Recognizing atrial flutter

This rhythm strip illustrates atrial flutter.

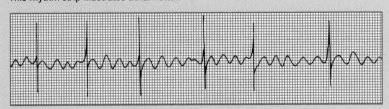

+ *Rhythm:* atrial — regular; ventricular — typically irregular
+ *Rate:* atrial — 280 beats/minute; ventricular — 60 beats/minute; ventricular rate depends on degree of atrioventricular block
+ *P wave:* classic sawtooth appearance referred to as flutter or F waves

+ *PR interval:* unmeasurable
+ *QRS complex:* 0.08 second; duration usually normal
+ *T wave:* unidentifiable
+ *QT interval:* unmeasurable
+ *Other:* atrial rate — greater than the ventricular rate

encountered in patients following cardiac surgery or in patients with acute myocardial infarction, chronic pulmonary disease, or systemic arterial hypoxia. Atrial flutter rarely occurs in healthy people. When it does, it may indicate intrinsic cardiac disease.

CLINICAL SIGNIFICANCE

The clinical significance of atrial flutter is determined by the number of impulses conducted through the atrioventricular (AV) node. That number is expressed as a conduction ratio, such as 2:1 or 4:1, and the resulting ventricular rate. If the ventricular rate is too slow (below 40 beats/minute) or too fast (above 150 beats/minute), cardiac output can be seriously compromised.

Usually the faster the ventricular rate, the more dangerous the arrhythmia. Rapid ventricular rates reduce ventricular filling time and coronary perfusion, which can cause angina, heart failure, pulmonary edema, hypotension, and syncope.

ECG CHARACTERISTICS

✦ *Rhythm:* Atrial rhythm is regular. Ventricular rhythm depends on the AV conduction pattern; it's typically regular, although cycles may alternate. An irregular pattern may signal atrial fibrillation or indicate development of a block.

✦ *Rate:* Atrial rate is 250 to 400 beats/minute. Ventricular rate depends on the degree of AV block; usually it's 60 to 100 beats/minute, but it may accelerate to 125 to 150 beats/minute.

Varying degrees of AV block produce ventricular rates that are usually one-half to one-fourth of the atrial rate. These are expressed as ratios, for example, 2:1 or 4:1. Usually, the AV node won't accept more than 180 impulses/minute and allows every second, third, or fourth impulse to be conducted. These impulses account for the ventricular rate. At the time atrial flutter is initially recognized, the ventricular response is typically above 100 beats/minute. One of the most common ventricular rates is 150 beats/minute with an atrial rate of 300, known as 2:1 block.

✦ *P wave:* Atrial flutter is characterized by abnormal P waves that produce a sawtooth appearance, referred to as flutter or F waves.

✦ *PR interval:* Unmeasurable.

✦ *QRS complex:* Duration is usually within normal limits, but the complex may be widened if flutter waves are buried within the complex.

✦ *T wave:* Not identifiable.

✦ *QT interval:* Unmeasurable because the T wave isn't identifiable.

✦ *Other*: The patient may develop an atrial rhythm that commonly varies between a fibrillatory line and flutter waves. This variation is referred to as *atrial fib-flutter.* The ventricular response is irregular. At times it may be diffi-

ECG characteristics

✦ *Rhythm*—atrial rhythm regular; ventricular rhythm depends on AV conduction pattern
✦ *Rate*—atrial rate 250 to 400 beats/minute; ventricular rate depends on degree of AV block
✦ Common ventricular rate is 150 beats/minute with atrial rate of 300 (2:1 block)
✦ *P wave*—abnormal, producing sawtooth appearance (F waves)
✦ *QRS complex*—duration usually within normal limits

Distinguishing atrial flutter from atrial fibrillation

It isn't uncommon to see atrial flutter that has an irregular pattern of impulse conduction to the ventricles. In some leads, this may be confused with atrial fibrillation. Here's how to tell the two arrhythmias apart.

ATRIAL FLUTTER
- ◆ Look for characteristic abnormal P waves that produce a sawtooth appearance, referred to as flutter waves, or F waves. These can best be identified in leads I, II, and V_1.
- ◆ Remember that the atrial rhythm is regular. You should be able to map the F waves across the rhythm strip. While some F waves may occur within the QRS or T waves, subsequent F waves will be visible and occur on time.

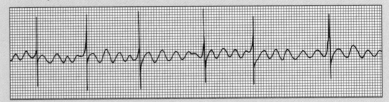

ATRIAL FIBRILLATION
- ◆ Fibrillatory or f waves occur in an irregular pattern, making the atrial rhythm irregular.
- ◆ If you identify atrial activity that at times looks like flutter waves and seems to be regular for a short time, and in other places the rhythm strip contains fibrillatory waves, interpret the rhythm as atrial fibrillation. Coarse fibrillatory waves may intermittently look similar to the characteristic sawtooth appearance of flutter waves.

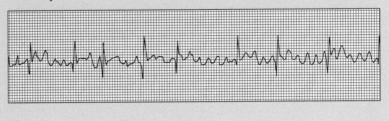

cult to distinguish atrial flutter from atrial fibrillation. (See *Distinguishing atrial flutter from atrial fibrillation.*)

SIGNS AND SYMPTOMS

When caring for a patient with atrial flutter, you may note that the peripheral and apical pulses are normal in rate and rhythm. That's because the pulse re-

Signs and symptoms
- ◆ Asymptomatic, if ventricular rate is normal
- ◆ Palpitations and signs and symptoms of reduced cardiac output, if ventricular rate is rapid

flects the number of ventricular contractions, not the number of atrial impulses.

If the ventricular rate is normal, the patient may be asymptomatic. If the ventricular rate is rapid, however, the patient may experience a feeling of palpitations and may exhibit signs and symptoms of reduced cardiac output.

INTERVENTIONS

If the patient is hemodynamically unstable, synchronized electrical cardioversion or countershock should be administered immediately. Cardioversion delivers electrical current to the heart to correct an arrhythmia, but unlike defibrillation, it usually uses much lower energy levels and is synchronized to discharge at the peak of the R wave. This causes immediate depolarization, interrupting reentry circuits and allowing the sinoatrial (SA) node to resume control as pacemaker. Synchronizing the energy current delivery with the R wave ensures that the current won't be delivered on the vulnerable T wave, which could initiate ventricular tachycardia or ventricular fibrillation.

The focus of treatment for hemodynamically stable patients with atrial flutter includes controlling the rate and converting the rhythm. Specific interventions depend on the patient's cardiac function, whether preexcitation syndromes are involved, and the duration (less than or greater than 48 hours) of the arrhythmia. For example, in atrial flutter with normal cardiac function and duration of rhythm less than 48 hours, electrical cardioversion may be considered; for duration greater than 48 hours, *don't use electrical cardioversion* because it increases the risk of thromboembolism unless the patient has been adequately anticoagulated.

Because atrial flutter may be an indication of intrinsic cardiac disease, monitor the patient closely for signs and symptoms of low cardiac output. Be alert to the effects of digoxin, which depresses the SA node.

If electrical cardioversion is indicated, prepare the patient for I.V. administration of a sedative or anesthetic as ordered. Keep resuscitative equipment at the bedside. Be alert for bradycardia because cardioversion can decrease the heart rate.

ATRIAL FIBRILLATION

Atrial fibrillation, sometimes called *AFib,* is defined as chaotic, asynchronous, electrical activity in atrial tissue. It results from the firing of multiple impulses from numerous ectopic pacemakers in the atria. Atrial fibrillation is characterized by the absence of P waves and an irregularly irregular ventricular response.

Interventions

Hemodynamically unstable
+ Immediate synchronized electrical cardioversion or countershock

Hemodynamically stable
+ Controlling rate and converting rhythm
+ Treatment depends on cardiac function (whether preexcitation syndromes are involved) and duration (< or > 48 hours)
+ Electrical cardioversion (with normal cardiac function, duration of rhythm < 48 hours)
+ Electrical cardioversion contraindicated (if duration > 48 hours due to increased risk of thromboembolism, unless adequately anticoagulated)

Atrial fibrillation
+ Chaotic, asynchronous, electrical activity in atrial tissue
+ Firing of multiple impulses from numerous ectopic pacemakers in atria

Atrial fibrillation
(continued)

+ Characterized by absence of P waves and irregular ventricular response
+ Considered controlled, when ventricular response rate drops below 100
+ Considered uncontrolled, when ventricular rate exceeds 100
+ Loss of atrial kick (like atrial flutter)

Causes

+ Cardiac surgery
+ Rheumatic heart disease
+ Valvular heart disease (especially mitral valve disease)
+ Hyperthyroidism
+ Pericarditis
+ CAD

When a number of ectopic sites in the atria initiate impulses, depolarization can't spread in an organized manner. Small sections of the atria are depolarized individually, resulting in the atrial muscle quivering instead of contracting. On an ECG, uneven baseline fibrillatory waves, or *f* waves, appear rather than clearly distinguishable P waves.

The atrioventricular (AV) node protects the ventricles from the 400 to 600 erratic atrial impulses that occur each minute by acting as a filter and blocking some of the impulses. The ventricles respond only to impulses conducted through the AV node, hence the characteristic, wide variation in R-R intervals. When the ventricular response rate drops below 100, atrial fibrillation is considered controlled. When the ventricular rate exceeds 100, the rhythm is considered uncontrolled. Atrial fibrillation is considered fast or uncontrolled at rates greater than 100. A "normal" ventricular response is defined as 60 to 100 beats/minute, so a ventricular rate of 100 is considered within normal.

Like atrial flutter, atrial fibrillation results in a loss of atrial kick. The rhythm may be sustained or paroxysmal, meaning that it occurs suddenly and ends abruptly. It can either be preceded by or be the result of premature atrial contractions. (See *Recognizing atrial fibrillation*.)

CAUSES

Atrial fibrillation occurs more commonly than atrial flutter or atrial tachycardia. Atrial fibrillation can occur following cardiac surgery. Other causes of atrial fibrillation include rheumatic heart disease, valvular heart disease (especially mitral valve disease), hyperthyroidism, pericarditis, coronary artery

---

Recognizing atrial fibrillation

This rhythm strip illustrates atrial fibrillation.

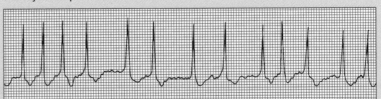

+ *Rhythm:* irregularly irregular
+ *Rate:* atrial — indiscernible; ventricular — 130 beats/minute
+ *P wave:* absent; replaced by fine fibrillatory waves, or f waves
+ *PR interval:* indiscernible
+ *QRS complex:* 0.08 second; duration and configuration are usually normal
+ *T wave:* indiscernible
+ *QT interval:* unmeasurable
+ *Other:* none

disease (CAD), acute myocardial infarction (MI), hypertension, cardiomyopathy, atrial septal defects, and chronic obstructive pulmonary disease.

The rhythm may also occur in a healthy person who smokes or drinks coffee or alcohol or who is fatigued and under stress. Certain drugs, such as aminophylline and digoxin, may contribute to the development of atrial fibrillation. Endogenous catecholamine released during exercise may also trigger the arrhythmia.

CLINICAL SIGNIFICANCE

The loss of atrial kick from atrial fibrillation can result in the subsequent loss of approximately 20% of normal end-diastolic volume. Combined with the decreased diastolic filling time associated with a rapid heart rate, clinically significant reductions in cardiac output can result. In uncontrolled atrial fibrillation, the patient may develop heart failure, myocardial ischemia, or syncope.

Patients with preexisting cardiac disease, such as hypertrophic cardiomyopathy, mitral stenosis, rheumatic heart disease, or those with mitral prosthetic valves, tend to tolerate atrial fibrillation poorly and may develop severe heart failure.

Left untreated, atrial fibrillation can lead to cardiovascular collapse, thrombus formation, and systemic arterial or pulmonary embolism. (See *Risk of restoring sinus rhythm.*)

ECG CHARACTERISTICS

✦ *Rhythm:* Atrial and ventricular rhythms are grossly irregular, typically described as irregularly irregular.
✦ *Rate:* The atrial rate is almost indiscernible and usually exceeds 400 beats/minute. The atrial rate far exceeds the ventricular rate because most impulses aren't conducted through the AV junction. The ventricular rate usually

Causes
(continued)
✦ Acute MI
✦ Hypertension
✦ Cardiomyopathy
✦ Atrial septal defects
✦ COPD
✦ Cigarettes, coffee, alcohol, fatigue, stress (in otherwise healthy person)
✦ Drugs (aminophylline, digoxin)

ECG characteristics
✦ *Rhythm*—atrial and ventricular rhythms irregularly irregular
✦ *Rate*—atrial rate barely discernible, usually exceeds 400 beats/minute; ventricular rate varies

---

Risk of restoring sinus rhythm

A patient with atrial fibrillation is at increased risk for developing atrial thrombus and subsequent systemic arterial embolism. In atrial fibrillation, neither atrium contracts as a whole. As a result, blood may pool on the atrial wall, and thrombi may form. Thrombus formation places the patient at higher risk for emboli and stroke.

If normal sinus rhythm is restored and the atria contract normally, clots may break away from the atrial wall and travel through the pulmonary or systemic circulation with potentially disastrous results, such as stroke, pulmonary embolism, or arterial occlusion.

ECG characteristics
(continued)

+ *P wave*—absent; erratic baseline F waves appear
+ *PR interval*—indiscernible
+ *QRS complex*—duration and configuration usually normal

Signs and symptoms

+ Pulse rate is irregularly irregular
+ Signs and symptoms of decreased cardiac output including hypotension and light-headedness (new onset of atrial fibrillation)
+ Possibly asymptomatic (chronic atrial fibrillation); however, face increased risk of pulmonary, cerebral, or other thromboembolic events

Interventions

+ Focus on reducing ventricular response rate to < 100 beats/minute
+ Immediate synchronized cardioversion (if hemodynamically unstable); most successful within 48 hours after onset

varies, typically from 100 to 150 beats/minute but can be below 100 beats/minute.

+ *P wave:* The P wave is absent. Erratic baseline F waves appear in place of P waves. These chaotic waves represent atrial tetanization from rapid atrial depolarizations.
+ *PR interval:* Indiscernible.
+ *QRS complex:* Duration and configuration are usually normal.
+ *T wave:* Indiscernible.
+ *QT interval:* Unmeasurable.
+ *Other:* The patient may develop an atrial rhythm that commonly varies between a fibrillatory line and flutter waves, a phenomenon called *atrial fib-flutter.* At times it may be difficult to distinguish atrial fibrillation from multifocal atrial tachycardia and from junctional rhythm. (*See Distinguishing atrial fibrillation from multifocal atrial tachycardia.* Also see *Distinguishing atrial fibrillation from junctional rhythm,* page 86.)

SIGNS AND SYMPTOMS

When caring for a patient with atrial fibrillation, you may find that the radial pulse rate is slower than the apical rate. The weaker contractions that occur in atrial fibrillation don't produce a palpable peripheral pulse; only the stronger ones do.

The pulse rhythm will be irregularly irregular, with a normal or abnormal heart rate. Patients with a new onset of atrial fibrillation and a rapid ventricular rate may demonstrate signs and symptoms of decreased cardiac output, including hypotension and light-headedness. Patients with chronic atrial fibrillation may be able to compensate for the decreased cardiac output. Although these patients may be asymptomatic, they face a greater-than-normal risk of the development of pulmonary, cerebral, or other thromboembolic events.

INTERVENTIONS

Treatment of atrial fibrillation aims to reduce the ventricular response rate to below 100 beats/minute. This may be accomplished either by drugs that control the ventricular response or by a combination of electrical cardioversion and drug therapy, to convert the arrhythmia to normal sinus rhythm. When the onset of atrial fibrillation is acute and the patient can cooperate, vagal maneuvers or carotid sinus massage may slow the ventricular response but won't convert the arrhythmia.

If the patient is hemodynamically unstable, synchronized electrical cardioversion should be administered immediately. Electrical cardioversion is most successful if used within the first 48 hours after onset and less successful the longer the duration of the arrhythmia. Conversion to normal sinus

Distinguishing atrial fibrillation from multifocal atrial tachycardia

To help you determine whether a rhythm is atrial fibrillation or the similar multifocal atrial tachycardia (MAT), focus on the presence of P waves as well as the atrial and ventricular rhythms. You may find it helpful to look at a longer (greater than 6 seconds) rhythm strip.

ATRIAL FIBRILLATION
✦ Carefully look for discernible P waves before each QRS complex.
✦ If you can't clearly identify P waves, and fibrillatory waves, or f waves, appear in the place of P waves, then the rhythm is probably atrial fibrillation.
✦ Carefully look at the rhythm, focusing on the R-R intervals. Remember that one of the hallmarks of atrial fibrillation is an irregularly irregular rhythm.

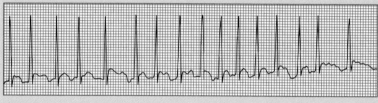

MAT
✦ P waves are present in MAT. Keep in mind, though, that the shape of the P waves will vary, with at least three different P wave shapes visible in a single rhythm strip.
✦ You should be able to see most, if not all, the various P wave shapes repeat.
✦ Although the atrial and ventricular rhythms are irregular, the irregularity generally isn't as pronounced as in atrial fibrillation.

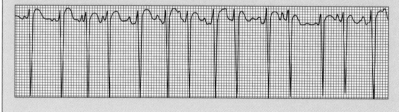

rhythm will cause forceful atrial contractions to resume abruptly. If a thrombus forms in the atria, the resumption of contractions can result in systemic emboli. (See *How synchronized cardioversion works,* page 87.)

The focus of treatment for hemodynamically stable patients with atrial fibrillation includes controlling the rate, converting the rhythm, and providing anticoagulation if indicated. Specific interventions depend on the patient's cardiac function, whether preexcitation syndromes are involved, and the duration of the arrhythmia.

Interventions
(continued)
✦ Control rate, convert rhythm, and provide anticoagulation, if indicated (if hemodynamically stable)

LOOK-ALIKES

Distinguishing atrial fibrillation from junctional rhythm

At times, it can be easy to mistake atrial fibrillation for junctional rhythm. Here's how to tell the two apart.

ATRIAL FIBRILLATION
✦ Examine lead II, which provides a clear view of atrial activity. Look for fibrillatory waves, or f waves, which appear as a wavy line. These waves indicate atrial fibrillation.
✦ Chronic atrial fibrillation tends to have fine or small f waves and a controlled ventricular rate (below 100 beats/minute).

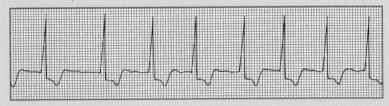

JUNCTIONAL RHYTHM
✦ In lead II, if you can find inverted P waves after or within 0.12 second before the QRS complex (see shaded area below), the rhythm is junctional.

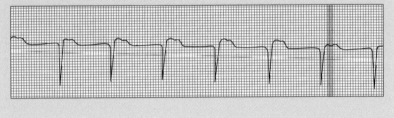

Interventions
(continued)
✦ Beta-adrenergic blockers and calcium channel blockers to control ventricular rate
✦ Anticoagulation to reduce risk of thromboembolism

Beta-adrenergic blockers and calcium channel blockers are the drugs of choice to control the ventricular rate. Patients with reduced left ventricular function typically receive digoxin. Anticoagulation is crucial in reducing the risk of thromboembolism. Heparin and warfarin are used for anticoagulation and to prepare the patient for electrical cardioversion. Symptomatic atrial fibrillation that doesn't respond to routine treatment may be treated with radiofrequency ablation therapy.

When assessing a patient with atrial fibrillation, assess the peripheral and apical pulses. If the patient isn't on a cardiac monitor, be alert for an irregular pulse and differences in the radial and apical pulse rates.

Assess for symptoms of decreased cardiac output and heart failure. If drug therapy is used, monitor serum drug levels and observe the patient for evi-

How synchronized cardioversion works

A patient experiencing an arrhythmia that leads to reduced cardiac output may be a candidate for synchronized cardioversion. This procedure may be done electively or as an emergency. For example, it may be an elective procedure in a patient with recurrent atrial fibrillation or an emergency procedure in a patient with ventricular tachycardia and a pulse.

Synchronized cardioversion is similar to defibrillation, also called *unsynchronized cardioversion,* except that synchronized cardioversion generally requires lower energy levels. Synchronizing the energy delivered to the patient reduces the risk that the current will strike during the relative refractory period of a cardiac cycle and induce ventricular fibrillation (VF).

In synchronized cardioversion, the R wave on the patient's electrocardiogram is synchronized with the cardioverter (defibrillator). After the firing buttons have been pressed, the cardioverter discharges energy when it senses the next R wave.

Keep in mind that a slight delay occurs between the time the discharge buttons are depressed and the moment the energy is actually discharged. When using handheld paddles, continue to hold the paddles on the patient's chest until the energy is delivered.

Remember to reset the "sync mode" on the defibrillator after each synchronized cardioversion. Resetting this switch is necessary because most defibrillators will automatically reset to an unsynchronized mode.

If VF occurs during the procedure, turn off the sync button and immediately deliver an unsynchronized defibrillation to terminate the arrhythmia. Be aware that synchronized cardioversion carries the risk of lethal arrhythmia when used in patients with digoxin toxicity.

Understanding synchronized cardioversion

+ R wave on ECG is synchronized with cardioverter
+ After pressing firing buttons, cardioverter discharges energy when it senses next R wave
+ Reset "sync mode" after each synchronized cardioversion
+ If VF occurs, turn off sync button and promptly deliver unsynchronized defibrillation

dence of toxicity. Tell the patient to report pulse rate changes, syncope or dizziness, chest pain, and signs of heart failure, such as dyspnea and peripheral edema.

ASHMAN'S PHENOMENON

Ashman's phenomenon refers to the aberrant conduction of premature supraventricular beats to the ventricles. (See *Ashman's phenomenon,* page 88.) This benign phenomenon is frequently associated with atrial fibrillation but can occur with any arrhythmia that affects the R-R interval.

CAUSES

Ashman's phenomenon is caused by a prolonged refractory period associated with slower rhythms. In theory, a conduction aberration occurs when a short cycle follows a long cycle because the refractory period varies with the length

Ashman's phenomenon

+ Aberrant conduction of premature supraventricular beats to ventricles
+ Frequently associated with atrial fibrillation

Causes

+ Prolonged refractory period associated with slower rhythms

Ashman's phenomenon

This rhythm strip illustrates Ashman's phenomenon.

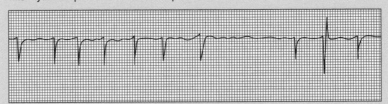

+ *Rhythm:* atrial and ventricular — irregular
+ *Rate:* underlying rhythm of 90 beats/minute
+ *P wave:* absent; fibrillatory waves
+ *PR interval:* not measurable

+ *QRS complex:* 0.12 second; right bundle-branch block (RBBB) pattern present on Ashman beat
+ *T wave:* deflection opposite that of QRS complex in the Ashman beat
+ *QT interval:* usually changed due to RBBB
+ *Other:* no compensatory pause after the aberrant beat; aberrancy may continue for several beats

of the cycle. An impulse that ends a short cycle preceded by a long one is more likely to reach refractory tissue.

The normal refractory period for the right bundle branch is slightly longer than the left one, so premature beats frequently reach the right bundle when it's partially or completely refractory. Because of this tendency, the abnormal beat is usually seen as a right bundle-branch block (RBBB).

CLINICAL SIGNIFICANCE

The importance of recognizing aberrantly conducted beats is primarily to prevent misdiagnosis and subsequent mistaken treatment of ventricular ectopy.

ECG CHARACTERISTICS

+ *Rhythm:* Atrial and ventricular rhythms are irregular.
+ *Rate:* Atrial and ventricular rates reflect the underlying rhythm.
+ *P wave:* The P wave has an abnormal configuration. It may be visible. If present in the underlying rhythm, the P wave is unchanged.
+ *PR interval:* If measurable, the interval often changes on the premature beat.

ECG characteristics

+ *Rhythm*—atrial and ventricular rhythms irregular
+ *Rate*—atrial and ventricular rates reflect underlying rhythm
+ *P wave*—abnormal configuration

✦ *QRS complex:* Configuration is usually altered, revealing an RBBB pattern.

✦ *T wave:* Deflection opposite that of the QRS complex occurs in most leads as a result of RBBB.

✦ *QT interval:* Usually has changed as a result of the RBBB.

✦ *Other:* There's no compensatory pause after an aberrant beat. The aberrancy may continue for several beats and typically ends a short cycle preceded by a long cycle.

SIGNS AND SYMPTOMS

No signs and symptoms related to this phenomenon.

INTERVENTIONS

None needed for this phenomenon.

WANDERING PACEMAKER

Wandering pacemaker, also called *wandering atrial pacemaker*, is an atrial arrhythmia that results when the site of impulse formation shifts from the sinoatrial (SA) node to another area above the ventricles. The origin of the impulse may wander beat to beat from the SA node to ectopic sites in the atria or to the atrioventricular (AV) junctional tissue. The P wave and PR interval vary from beat to beat as the pacemaker site changes. (See *Recognizing wandering pacemaker.*)

Recognizing wandering pacemaker

This rhythm strip illustrates wandering pacemaker.

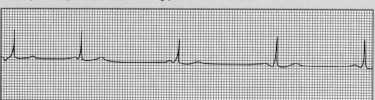

✦ *Rhythm:* atrial and ventricular — irregular

✦ *Rate:* atrial and ventricular — 50 beats/minute

✦ *P wave:* changes in size and shape; first P wave inverted, second upright

✦ *PR interval:* varied

✦ *QRS complex:* 0.08 second

✦ *T wave:* normal

✦ *QT interval:* 0.44 second

✦ *Other:* none

ECG characteristics
(continued)

✦ *QRS complex*—configuration usually altered, revealing RBBB pattern

✦ *T wave*—deflection opposite (that of QRS complex) as a result of RBBB

✦ *Other*—no compensatory pause after aberrant beat

Wandering pacemaker

✦ Atrial arrhythmia that results when site of impulse formation shifts from SA node to an area above ventricles

✦ Impulse may wander beat to beat from SA node to ectopic sites in atria or to AV junctional tissue

Causes

+ Increased parasympathetic (vagal) influences on SA node or AV junction
+ Chronic pulmonary disease
+ Valvular heart disease
+ Digoxin toxicity
+ Inflammation of atrial tissue

ECG characteristics

+ *Rhythm*—atrial and ventricular rhythms vary
+ *Rate*—atrial and ventricular rates vary, but usually within normal limits
+ *P wave*—altered size and configuration (at least three different shapes visible)
+ *PR interval*—varies from beat to beat as pacemaker site changes
+ *QRS complex*—usually within normal limits with normal configuration

Signs and symptoms

+ Generally asymptomatic

CAUSES

In most cases, wandering pacemaker is caused by increased parasympathetic (vagal) influences on the SA node or AV junction. It can also be caused by chronic pulmonary disease, valvular heart disease, digoxin toxicity, and inflammation of the atrial tissue.

CLINICAL SIGNIFICANCE

The arrhythmia may be normal in young patients and is common in athletes who have slow heart rates. The arrhythmia may be difficult to identify because it's often transient. Although wandering pacemaker is rarely serious, chronic arrhythmias are a sign of heart disease and should be monitored.

ECG CHARACTERISTICS

+ *Rhythm:* The atrial rhythm varies slightly, with an irregular P-P interval. The ventricular rhythm varies slightly, with an irregular R-R interval.
+ *Rate:* Atrial and ventricular rates vary but are usually within normal limits, or below 60 beats/minute.
+ *P wave:* Altered size and configuration are due to the changing pacemaker site (SA node, atria, or AV junction). The P wave may also be absent, inverted, or may follow the QRS complex if the impulse originates in the AV junction. A combination of these variations may appear, with at least three different P-wave shapes visible.
+ *PR interval:* The PR interval varies from beat to beat as the pacemaker site changes but usually less than 0.20 second. If the impulse originates in the AV junction, the PR interval will be less than 0.12 second. This variation in PR interval will cause a slightly irregular R-R interval. When the P wave is present, the PR interval may be normal or shortened.
+ *QRS complex:* Ventricular depolarization is normal, so duration of the QRS complex is usually within normal limits and is of normal configuration.
+ *T wave:* Normal size and configuration.
+ *QT interval:* Usually within normal limits, but may vary.
+ *Other:* At times it may be difficult to distinguish wandering pacemaker from premature atrial contractions. (See *Distinguishing wandering pacemaker from premature atrial contractions.*)

SIGNS AND SYMPTOMS

Patients are generally asymptomatic and unaware of the arrhythmia. The pulse rate may be normal or below 60 beats/minute, and the rhythm may be regular or slightly irregular.

LOOK-ALIKES

Distinguishing wandering pacemaker from premature atrial contractions

Because premature atrial contractions (PACs) are commonly encountered, it's possible to mistake wandering pacemaker for PACs unless the rhythm strip is carefully examined. In such cases, you may find it helpful to look at a longer (greater than 6 seconds) rhythm strip.

WANDERING PACEMAKER

+ Carefully examine the P waves. You must be able to identify at least three different shapes of P waves (see shaded areas below) in wandering pacemaker.
+ Atrial rhythm varies slightly, with an irregular P-P interval. Ventricular rhythm varies slightly, with an irregular R-R interval. These slight variations in rhythm result from the changing site of impulse formation.

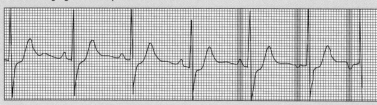

PAC

+ The PAC occurs earlier than the sinus P wave, with an abnormal configuration when compared with a sinus P wave (see shaded area below). It's possible, but rare, to see multifocal PACs, which originate from multiple ectopic pacemaker sites in the atria. In this setting, the P waves may have different shapes.
+ With the exception of the irregular atrial and ventricular rhythms as a result of the PAC, the underlying rhythm is usually regular.

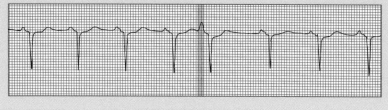

INTERVENTIONS

Usually, no treatment is needed for asymptomatic patients. If the patient is symptomatic, however, the patient's medications should be reviewed and the underlying cause investigated and treated. Monitor the patient's heart rhythm and assess for signs of hemodynamic instability, such as hypotension and changes in mental status.

Interventions

+ Unnecessary for asymptomatic patients
+ If symptomatic, focus on investigating and treating underlying cause

Junctional arrhythmias

Junctional arrhythmias originate in the atrioventricular (AV) junction—the area in and around the AV node and the bundle of His. The specialized pacemaker cells in the AV junction take over as the heart's pacemaker if the sinoatrial (SA) node fails to function properly or if the electrical impulses originating in the SA node are blocked. These junctional pacemaker cells have an inherent firing rate of 40 to 60 beats/minute.

In normal impulse conduction, the AV node slows transmission of the impulse from the atria to the ventricles, which allows the ventricles to fill as much as possible before they contract. However, these impulses don't always follow the normal conduction pathway. (See *Conduction in Wolff-Parkinson-White syndrome,* page 94.)

Because of the location of the AV junction within the conduction pathway, electrical impulses originating in this area cause abnormal depolarization of the heart. The impulse is conducted in a retrograde (backward) fashion to depolarize the atria, and antegrade (forward) to depolarize the ventricles.

Depolarization of the atria can precede depolarization of the ventricles, or the ventricles can be depolarized before the atria. Depolarization of the atria and ventricles can also occur simultaneously. (See *Locating the P wave,* page 95.)

Retrograde depolarization of the atria results in inverted P waves in leads II, III, and aV$_F$, leads in which you would normally see upright P waves appear.

Junctional arrhythmias

✦ Originate in AV junction (area in and around AV node and bundle of His)
✦ Specialized pacemaker cells in AV junction take over if SA node malfunctions
✦ Depolarization of atria can occur before that of ventricles or vice versa (depolarization of both can also occur at same time)
✦ Retrograde depolarization of atria results in inverted P waves in leads II, III, and aV$_F$

Conduction in Wolff-Parkinson-White syndrome

Electrical impulses in the heart don't always follow normal conduction pathways. In preexcitation syndromes, electrical impulses enter the ventricles from the atria through an accessory pathway that bypasses the atrioventricular junction. Wolff-Parkinson-White (WPW) syndrome is a common type of preexcitation syndrome.

WPW syndrome commonly occurs in young children and in adults ages 20 to 35. The syndrome causes the PR interval to shorten and the QRS complex to lengthen as a result of a delta wave. Delta waves, which in WPW occur just before normal ventricular depolarization, are produced as a result of the premature depolarization or preexcitation of a portion of the ventricles.

WPW is clinically significant because the accessory pathway — in this case, Kent's bundle — may result in paroxysmal tachyarrhythmias by reentry and rapid conduction mechanisms.

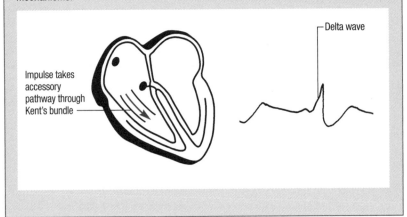

Impulse takes accessory pathway through Kent's bundle

Delta wave

Junctional arrhythmias
(continued)

✦ Atrial sometimes mistaken for junctional because impulses are generated so low in atria, causing retrograde atrial depolarization and inverted P waves

Originating in atria
✦ Arrhythmia with inverted P wave before QRS complex with normal PR interval (0.12 to 0.20 second)

Originating in AV junction
✦ Arrhythmia with PR interval < 0.12 second

Keep in mind that arrhythmias causing inverted P waves on an ECG may originate in the atria or AV junction. Atrial arrhythmias are sometimes mistaken for junctional arrhythmias because impulses are generated so low in the atria that they cause retrograde depolarization and inverted P waves. Looking at the PR interval will help you determine whether an arrhythmia is atrial or junctional.

An arrhythmia with an inverted P wave before the QRS complex and with a normal PR interval (0.12 to 0.20 second) originates in the atria. An arrhythmia with a PR interval less than 0.12 second originates in the AV junction.

KNOW-HOW

Locating the P wave

When the specialized pacemaker cells in the atrioventricular junction take over as the dominant pacemaker of the heart:
+ depolarization of the atria can precede depolarization of the ventricles
+ the ventricles can be depolarized before the atria
+ simultaneous depolarization of the atria and ventricles can occur.

The rhythm strips shown here demonstrate the various locations of the P waves in junctional arrhythmias, depending on the direction of depolarization.

INVERTED P WAVE
If the atria are depolarized first, the P wave will occur before the QRS complex.

INVERTED P WAVE
If the ventricles are depolarized first, the P wave will occur after the QRS complex.

INVERTED P WAVE (HIDDEN)
If the ventricles and atria are depolarized simultaneously, the P wave will be hidden in the QRS complex.

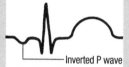
Inverted P wave

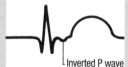
Inverted P wave

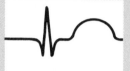

PREMATURE JUNCTIONAL CONTRACTIONS

A premature junctional contraction (PJC) is a junctional beat that occurs before a normal sinus beat; it interrupts the underlying rhythm and causes an irregular rhythm. These ectopic beats commonly occur as a result of enhanced automaticity in the junctional tissue or bundle of His. As with all impulses generated in the atrioventricular (AV) junction, the atria are depolarized in a retrograde fashion, causing an inverted P wave. The ventricles are depolarized normally. (See *Recognizing a PJC,* page 96.)

CAUSES

PJCs may be caused by digoxin toxicity, excessive caffeine intake, amphetamine ingestion, excessive alcohol intake, excessive nicotine intake, stress, coronary artery disease, myocardial ischemia, valvular heart disease, peri-

PJCs
+ Junctional beat that occurs before normal sinus beat, causing irregular rhythm

Causes
+ Digoxin toxicity
+ Excessive caffeine, alcohol, or nicotine
+ Amphetamines
+ Stress
+ CAD, myocardial ischemia, valvular heart disease, pericarditis, or heart failure

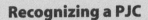

Recognizing a PJC

This rhythm strip illustrates sinus rhythm with premature junctional contractions (PJCs).

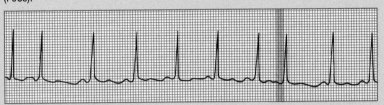

- ✦ *Rhythm:* irregular atrial and ventricular rhythms during PJCs
- ✦ *Rate:* 100 beats/minute
- ✦ *P wave:* inverted and precedes the QRS complex (see shaded area)
- ✦ *PR interval:* 0.14 second for the underlying rhythm and 0.06 second for the PJC
- ✦ *QRS complex:* 0.06 second
- ✦ *T wave:* normal configuration
- ✦ *QT interval:* 0.36 second
- ✦ *Other:* compensatory pause may follow PJCs

Causes
(continued)

- ✦ COPD
- ✦ Hyperthyroidism
- ✦ Electrolyte imbalances
- ✦ Inflammatory changes in AV junction

ECG characteristics

- ✦ *Rhythm*—atrial and ventricular rhythms irregular (underlying rhythm may be regular)
- ✦ *Rate*—reflects underlying rhythm
- ✦ *P wave*—may occur before or after QRS complex or may appear absent when hidden in the QRS complex

carditis, heart failure, chronic obstructive pulmonary disease (COPD), hyperthyroidism, electrolyte imbalances, or inflammatory changes in the AV junction after heart surgery.

CLINICAL SIGNIFICANCE

PJCs are generally considered harmless unless they occur frequently—typically defined as more than six per minute. Frequent PJCs indicate junctional irritability and can precipitate a more serious arrhythmia, such as junctional tachycardia. In patients taking digoxin, PJCs are a common early sign of toxicity.

ECG CHARACTERISTICS

Rhythm: Atrial and ventricular rhythms are irregular during PJCs; the underlying rhythm may be regular.

Rate: Atrial and ventricular rates reflect the underlying rhythm.

P wave: The P wave is usually inverted. It may occur before or after the QRS complex or may appear absent when hidden in the QRS complex. Look for an inverted P wave in leads II, III, and aV$_F$. Depending on the initial direction of depolarization, the P wave may fall before, during, or after the QRS complex.

PR interval: If the P wave precedes the QRS complex, the PR interval is shortened (less than 0.12 second); otherwise, it can't be measured.

QRS complex: Because the ventricles are usually depolarized normally, the QRS complex usually has a normal configuration and a normal duration of less than 0.12 second.

T wave: Usually has a normal configuration.

QT interval: Usually within normal limits.

Other: A compensatory pause reflecting retrograde atrial conduction may follow the PJC.

SIGNS AND SYMPTOMS

The patient is usually asymptomatic. He may complain of palpitations or a feeling of "skipped heart beats." You may be able to palpate an irregular pulse when PJCs occur. If PJCs are frequent enough, the patient may experience hypotension from a transient decrease in cardiac output.

INTERVENTIONS

PJCs don't usually require treatment unless the patient is symptomatic. In those cases, the underlying cause should be treated. For example, in digoxin toxicity, the medication should be discontinued and serum drug levels monitored.

Monitor the patient for hemodynamic instability as well. If ectopic beats occur frequently, the patient should decrease or eliminate his caffeine intake.

JUNCTIONAL ESCAPE RHYTHM

A junctional escape rhythm, also referred to as *junctional rhythm,* is an arrhythmia originating in the atrioventricular (AV) junction. In this arrhythmia, the AV junction takes over as a secondary, or "escape" pacemaker. This usually occurs only when a higher pacemaker site in the atria, usually the sinoatrial (SA) node, fails as the heart's dominant pacemaker.

Remember that the AV junction can take over as the heart's dominant pacemaker if the firing rate of the higher pacemaker sites falls below the AV junction's intrinsic firing rate, if the pacemaker fails to generate an impulse, or if the conduction of the impulses is blocked.

ECG characteristics
(continued)

+ *PR interval*—shortened (< 0.12 second) if P wave precedes QRS complex
+ *QRS complex*—within normal limits

Signs and symptoms

+ Asymptomatic (usually)
+ Palpitations
+ Irregular pulse (upon palpation)
+ Hypotension from transient decrease in cardiac output (if PJCs are frequent enough)

Interventions

+ Unneccesary in asymptomatic patients
+ Focus on underlying cause in symptomatic patients

Junctional escape rhythm

+ AV junction takes over as secondary pacemaker
+ Usually occurs when SA node fails as the dominant pacemaker
+ Atria are depolarized via retrograde conduction
+ P waves are inverted, and impulse conduction through ventricles is normal
+ Firing rate in AV junction is 40 to 60 beats/minute

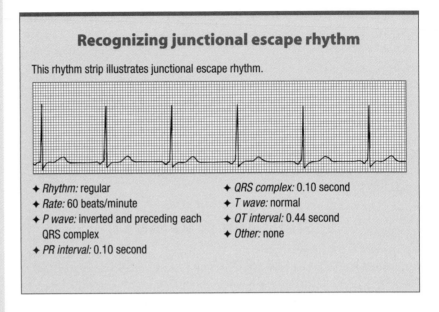

Recognizing junctional escape rhythm

This rhythm strip illustrates junctional escape rhythm.

+ *Rhythm:* regular
+ *Rate:* 60 beats/minute
+ *P wave:* inverted and preceding each QRS complex
+ *PR interval:* 0.10 second
+ *QRS complex:* 0.10 second
+ *T wave:* normal
+ *QT interval:* 0.44 second
+ *Other:* none

In a junctional escape rhythm, as in all junctional arrhythmias, the atria are depolarized by means of retrograde conduction. The P waves are inverted, and impulse conduction through the ventricles is normal. The normal intrinsic firing rate for cells in the AV junction is 40 to 60 beats/minute. (See *Recognizing junctional escape rhythm.*)

CAUSES

Causes

+ SA node ischemia
+ Hypoxia
+ Electrolyte imbalances
+ Valvular heart disease
+ Heart failure
+ Cardiomyopathy
+ Myocarditis
+ SSS
+ Increased parasympathetic tone
+ Drugs

A junctional escape rhythm can be caused by a condition that disturbs normal SA node function or impulse conduction. Causes of the arrhythmia include SA node ischemia, hypoxia, electrolyte imbalances, valvular heart disease, heart failure, cardiomyopathy, myocarditis, sick sinus syndrome (SSS), and increased parasympathetic (vagal) tone. Drugs, such as digoxin, calcium channel blockers, and beta-adrenergic blockers, can also cause a junctional escape rhythm.

CLINICAL SIGNIFICANCE

The clinical significance of junctional escape rhythm depends on how well the patient tolerates a decreased heart rate (40 to 60 beats/minute) and associated decrease in cardiac output. In addition to a decreased cardiac output from a slower heart rate, depolarization of the atria either after or simultaneously with ventricular depolarization results in loss of atrial kick. Remember that junctional escape rhythms protect the heart from potentially life-threatening ventricular escape rhythms.

ECG CHARACTERISTICS

Rhythm: Atrial and ventricular rhythms are regular.
Rate: The atrial and ventricular rates are 40 to 60 beats/minute.
P wave: The P wave is inverted (look for inverted P waves in leads II, III, and aV$_F$). The P wave may occur before or after the QRS complex or may appear absent when hidden within QRS complex.
PR interval: If the P wave precedes the QRS complex, the PR interval is shortened (less than 0.12 second); otherwise, it can't be measured.
QRS complex: Duration is usually within normal limits; configuration is usually normal.
T wave: Usually normal configuration.
QT interval: Usually within normal limits.
Other: None.

SIGNS AND SYMPTOMS

A patient with a junctional escape rhythm will have a slow, regular pulse rate of 40 to 60 beats/minute. The patient may be asymptomatic. However, pulse rates under 60 beats/minute may lead to inadequate cardiac output, causing hypotension, syncope, or blurred vision.

INTERVENTIONS

Treatment for a junctional escape rhythm involves identification and correction of the underlying cause, whenever possible. (See *Bradycardia algorithm,* page 53, in chapter 4.) If the patient is symptomatic, atropine may be used to increase the heart rate, or a temporary (transcutaneous or transvenous) or permanent pacemaker may be inserted. Because junctional escape rhythm can prevent ventricular standstill, it should never be suppressed.

Monitor the patient's serum digoxin and electrolyte levels and watch for signs of decreased cardiac output, such as hypotension, syncope, and blurred vision.

ECG characteristics

✦ *Rhythm*—atrial and ventricular rhythms regular
✦ *Rate*—atrial and ventricular rates are 40 to 60 beats/minute
✦ *P wave*—inverted; may occur before or after QRS complex or may appear absent when hidden within QRS complex
✦ *PR interval*—shortened (< 0.12 second), if P wave precedes QRS complex
✦ *QRS complex*—within normal limits

Signs and symptoms

✦ Slow, regular pulse rate (40 to 60 beats/minute)
✦ May be asymptomatic, but rates < 60 beats/minute may lead to inadequate cardiac output, hypotension, syncope, or blurred vision

Interventions

✦ Identify and correct underlying cause (when possible)
✦ If symptomatic, atropine may increase heart rate; or, temporary or permanent pacemaker may be inserted

Accelerated junctional rhythm

+ Called *accelerated* because it occurs at rate of 60 to 100 beats/minute
+ Atria are depolarized through retrograde conduction; ventricles are depolarized normally

Causes

+ Digoxin toxicity (common)
+ Electrolyte disturbances
+ Valvular heart disease
+ Rheumatic heart disease
+ Heart failure
+ Myocarditis
+ Cardiac surgery
+ Inferior- or posterior-wall MI

ACCELERATED JUNCTIONAL RHYTHM

An accelerated junctional rhythm is an arrhythmia that originates in the atrioventricular (AV) junction and is usually caused by enhanced automaticity of the AV junctional tissue. It's called *accelerated* because it occurs at a rate of 60 to 100 beats/minute, exceeding the inherent junctional escape rate of 40 to 60 beats/minute.

Because the rate is below 100 beats/minute, the arrhythmia isn't classified as junctional tachycardia. The atria are depolarized by means of retrograde conduction, and the ventricles are depolarized normally. (See *Recognizing accelerated junctional rhythm.*)

 AGE CHANGE Up to age three years, the AV nodal escape rhythm is 50 to 80 beats/minute. Consequently, a junctional rhythm is considered accelerated only when greater than 80 beats/minute in infants and toddlers.

CAUSES

Digoxin toxicity is a common cause of accelerated junctional rhythm. Other causes include electrolyte disturbances, valvular heart disease, rheumatic heart disease, heart failure, myocarditis, cardiac surgery, and inferior- or posterior-wall myocardial infarction.

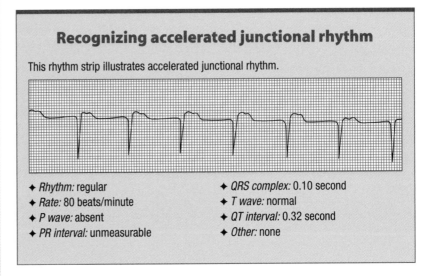

Recognizing accelerated junctional rhythm

This rhythm strip illustrates accelerated junctional rhythm.

+ *Rhythm:* regular
+ *Rate:* 80 beats/minute
+ *P wave:* absent
+ *PR interval:* unmeasurable
+ *QRS complex:* 0.10 second
+ *T wave:* normal
+ *QT interval:* 0.32 second
+ *Other:* none

CLINICAL SIGNIFICANCE

Patients experiencing accelerated junctional rhythm are generally asymptomatic because the rate corresponds to the normal inherent firing rate of the sinoatrial node (60 to 100 beats/minute). However, symptoms of decreased cardiac output, including hypotension and syncope, can occur if atrial depolarization occurs after or simultaneously with ventricular depolarization, which causes the subsequent loss of atrial kick.

ECG CHARACTERISTICS

Rhythm: Atrial and ventricular rhythms are regular.
Rate: Atrial and ventricular rates range from 60 to 100 beats/minute.
P wave: If the P wave is present, it will be inverted in leads II, III, and aV$_F$. It may precede, follow, or be hidden in the QRS complex.
PR interval: If the P wave occurs before the QRS complex, the PR interval is shortened (less than 0.12 second). Otherwise, it can't be measured.
QRS complex: Duration is usually within normal limits. Configuration is usually normal.
T wave: Usually within normal limits.
QT interval: Usually within normal limits.
Other: None.

Accelerated junctional rhythm can sometimes be difficult to distinguish from accelerated idioventricular rhythm. (See *Distinguishing accelerated idioventricular rhythm from accelerated junctional rhythm,* page 102.)

SIGNS AND SYMPTOMS

The pulse rate will be normal with a regular rhythm. The patient may be asymptomatic because accelerated junctional rhythm has the same rate as sinus rhythm. However, if cardiac output is decreased, the patient may exhibit symptoms, such as hypotension, changes in mental status, and weak peripheral pulses.

INTERVENTIONS

Treatment for accelerated junctional rhythm involves identifying and correcting the underlying cause. Assessing the patient for signs and symptoms related to decreased cardiac output and hemodynamic instability is key, as is monitoring serum digoxin and electrolyte levels.

ECG characteristics
+ *Rhythm*—atrial and ventricular rhythms regular
+ *Rate*—atrial and ventricular rates from 60 to 100 beats/minute
+ *P wave*—inverted in leads II, III, and aV$_F$; may precede, follow, or be hidden in QRS complex
+ *PR interval*—shortened (< 0.12 second), if P wave occurs before QRS complex
+ *QRS complex*—within normal limits

Signs and symptoms
+ May be asymptomatic because accelerated junctional rhythm has same rate as sinus rhythm
+ If cardiac output is decreased, symptoms include hypotension, changes in mental status, and weak peripheral pulses

Interventions
+ Identify and correct underlying cause
+ Assess for signs and symptoms related to decreased cardiac output and hemodynamic instability

LOOK-ALIKES

Distinguishing accelerated idioventricular rhythm from accelerated junctional rhythm

Accelerated idioventricular rhythm and accelerated junctional rhythm appear similar but have different causes. To distinguish between the two, closely examine the duration of the QRS complex and then look for P waves.

ACCELERATED IDIOVENTRICULAR RHYTHM
✦ The QRS duration will be greater than 0.12 second.
✦ The QRS will have a wide and bizarre configuration.
✦ P waves are usually absent.
✦ The ventricular rate is generally between 40 and 100 beats/minute.

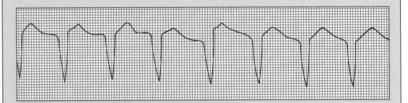

ACCELERATED JUNCTIONAL RHYTHM
✦ The QRS duration and configuration are usually normal.
✦ Inverted P waves generally occur before or after the QRS complex. However, remember that the P waves may also appear absent when hidden within the QRS complex.
✦ The ventricular rate is typically between 60 and 100 beats/minute.

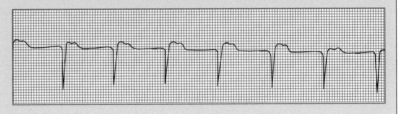

JUNCTIONAL TACHYCARDIA

In junctional tachycardia, three or more premature junctional contractions (PJCs) occur in a row. This supraventricular tachycardia generally occurs as a result of enhanced automaticity of the atrioventricular (AV) junction, which causes the AV junction to override the sinoatrial (SA) node as the dominant pacemaker.

In junctional tachycardia, the atria are depolarized by retrograde conduction. Conduction through the ventricles is normal. (See *Recognizing junctional tachycardia.*)

CAUSES

Digoxin toxicity is the most common cause of junctional tachycardia. In such cases, the arrhythmia can be aggravated by hypokalemia. Other causes of junctional tachycardia include inferior- or posterior-wall infarction or ischemia, inflammation of the AV junction after heart surgery, heart failure, electrolyte imbalances, and valvular heart disease.

Junctional tachycardia

✦ Three or more PJCs in a row
✦ AV junction overrides SA node as dominant pacemaker
✦ Atria are depolarized through retrograde conduction; conduction through ventricles is normal

Causes

✦ Digoxin toxicity (most common)
✦ Inferior- or posterior-wall infarction or ischemia
✦ Inflammation of AV junction after heart surgery
✦ Heart failure
✦ Electrolyte imbalances
✦ Valvular heart disease

Recognizing junctional tachycardia

This rhythm strip illustrates junctional tachycardia.

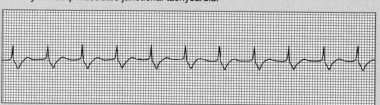

✦ *Rhythm:* atrial and ventricular — regular
✦ *Rate:* atrial and ventricular — 115 beats/minute
✦ *P wave:* inverted; follows QRS complex
✦ *PR interval:* unmeasurable
✦ *QRS complex:* 0.08 second
✦ *T wave:* normal
✦ *QT interval:* 0.36 second
✦ *Other:* none

CLINICAL SIGNIFICANCE

The clinical significance of junctional tachycardia depends on the rate and underlying cause. At higher ventricular rates, junctional tachycardia may reduce cardiac output by decreasing ventricular filling time. A loss of atrial kick also occurs with atrial depolarization that follows or occurs simultaneously with ventricular depolarization.

ECG characteristics

+ *Rhythm*—atrial and ventricular rhythms usually regular
+ *Rate*—atrial and ventricular rates > 100 beats/minute
+ *P wave*—usually inverted in leads II, III, and aV$_F$; may occur before or after QRS complex, or be hidden in QRS complex
+ *PR interval*—shortened (< 0.12 second), if P wave precedes QRS complex
+ *QRS complex*—within normal limits

ECG CHARACTERISTICS

Rhythm: Atrial and ventricular rhythms are usually regular. The atrial rhythm may be difficult to determine if the P wave is hidden in the QRS complex or preceding T wave.
Rate: Atrial and ventricular rates exceed 100 beats/minute (usually between 100 and 200 beats/minute). The atrial rate may be difficult to determine if the P wave is hidden in the QRS complex or the preceding T wave.
P wave: The P wave is usually inverted in leads II, III, and aV$_F$. It may occur before or after the QRS complex or be hidden in the QRS complex.
PR interval: If the P wave precedes the QRS complex, the PR interval is shortened (less than 0.12 second); otherwise, the PR interval can't be measured.
QRS complex: Duration is within normal limits; configuration is usually normal.
T wave: Configuration is usually normal but may be abnormal if the P wave is hidden in the T wave. The fast rate may make T waves indiscernible.
QT interval: Usually within normal limits.
Other: None.

Signs and symptoms

+ Pulse rate > 100 beats/minute, with regular rhythm
+ Hypotension, with decreased cardiac output and hemodynamic instability

SIGNS AND SYMPTOMS

The patient's pulse rate will be above 100 beats/minute and have a regular rhythm. Patients with a rapid heart rate may experience signs and symptoms of decreased cardiac output and hemodynamic instability including hypotension.

INTERVENTIONS

The underlying cause should be identified and treated. If the cause is digoxin toxicity, the drug should be discontinued. In some cases of digoxin toxicity, a digoxin-binding drug may be used to reduce serum digoxin levels. Vagal maneuvers and drugs, such as adenosine, may slow the heart rate for symptomatic patients. Patients with recurrent junctional tachycardia may be treated with ablation therapy, followed by permanent pacemaker insertion.

Monitor patients with junctional tachycardia for signs of decreased cardiac output. In addition, check digoxin and potassium levels and administer potassium supplements as ordered.

Interventions

+ Identify and treat underlying cause (for example, if digoxin is cause, must be discontinued)
+ Vagal maneuvers and drugs (adenosine) to slow heart rate in symptomatic patients
+ Ablation therapy followed by permanent pacemaker for recurrent tachycardia
+ Monitor for signs of decreased cardiac output

Ventricular arrhythmias

Ventricular arrhythmias originate in the ventricles below the bifurcation of the bundle of His. These arrhythmias occur when electrical impulses depolarize the myocardium using a different pathway from normal impulse conduction.

Ventricular arrhythmias appear on an ECG in characteristic ways. The QRS complex in most of these arrhythmias is wider than normal because of the prolonged conduction time through, and abnormal depolarization of, the ventricles. The deflections of the T wave and the QRS complex are in opposite directions because ventricular repolarization, as well as ventricular depolarization, is abnormal. The P wave in many ventricular arrhythmias is absent because atrial depolarization doesn't occur.

When electrical impulses come from the ventricles instead of the atria, atrial kick is lost and cardiac output can decrease by as much as 30%. This is one reason why patients with ventricular arrhythmias may show signs and symptoms of heart failure, including hypotension, angina, syncope, and respiratory distress.

Although ventricular arrhythmias may be benign, they're generally considered the most serious arrhythmias, because the ventricles are ultimately responsible for cardiac output. Rapid recognition and treatment of ventricular arrhythmias increases the chances of successful resuscitation.

Ventricular arrhythmias

+ Originate in ventricles below bifurcation of bundle of His
+ T wave and QRS complex (wider than normal) deflections are in opposite directions; P wave is usually absent
+ Atrial kick is lost and cardiac output decreased when electrical impulses come from ventricles versus atria
+ Most serious type of arrhythmia; rapid treatment increases chance for successful resuscitation

PVCs

+ Ectopic beats originating in ventricles, occurring earlier than expected
+ With underlying heart disease, may cause VT and VF
+ May occur singly, in pairs, or in clusters; may also appear in patterns (bigeminy, trigeminy)
+ May be *unifocal* (originate from same ventricular ectopic pacemaker site) or *multifocal* (originate from different ectopic pacemaker sites)

PREMATURE VENTRICULAR CONTRACTIONS

Premature ventricular contractions (PVCs) are ectopic beats that originate in the ventricles, occur earlier than expected. PVCs may occur in healthy people without being clinically significant.

When PVCs occur in patients with underlying heart disease, however, they may herald the development of lethal ventricular arrhythmias, including ventricular tachycardia (VT) and ventricular fibrillation (VF).

PVCs may occur singly, in pairs (couplets), or in clusters. PVCs may also appear in patterns, such as bigeminy or trigeminy. (See *Recognizing PVCs*.)

In many cases, PVCs are followed by a compensatory pause. PVCs may be uniform in appearance, arising from a single ectopic ventricular pacemaker site, or multiform, originating from different sites or originating from a single pacemaker site but having QRS complexes that differ in size, shape, and direction.

PVCs may also be described as unifocal or multifocal. Unifocal PVCs originate from the same ventricular ectopic pacemaker site, whereas multifocal PVCs originate from different ectopic pacemaker sites in the ventricles.

Recognizing PVCs

This rhythm strip illustrates normal sinus rhythm with premature ventricular contractions (PVCs).

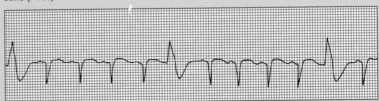

+ *Rhythm:* irregular
+ *Rate:* 120 beats/minute
+ *P wave:* none with PVC, but P wave present with other QRS complexes
+ *PR interval:* 0.12 second in underlying rhythm
+ *QRS complex:* early, with bizarre configuration and duration of 0.14 second

in PVC; QRS complexes are 0.08 second in underlying rhythm
+ *T wave:* normal; opposite direction from QRS complex
+ *QT interval:* 0.28 second with underlying rhythm
+ *Other:* none

CAUSES

PVCs are usually caused by enhanced automaticity in the ventricular conduction system or muscle tissue. The irritable focus results from a disruption of the normal electrolyte shifts during cellular depolarization and repolarization. Possible causes of PVCs include:

+ electrolyte imbalances, such as hypokalemia, hyperkalemia, hypomagnesemia, and hypocalcemia
+ metabolic acidosis
+ hypoxia
+ myocardial ischemia and infarction
+ drug intoxication, particularly with cocaine, amphetamines, digoxin, phenothiazines, and tricyclic antidepressants
+ enlargement or hypertrophy of the ventricular chambers
+ increased sympathetic stimulation
+ myocarditis
+ mitral valve prolapse
+ caffeine or alcohol ingestion
+ tobacco use
+ irritation of the ventricles by pacemaker electrodes or a pulmonary artery catheter
+ sympathomimetic drugs, such as epinephrine and isoproterenol.

CLINICAL SIGNIFICANCE

PVCs are significant for two reasons. First, they can lead to more serious arrhythmias, such as VT or VF. The risk of developing a more serious arrhythmia increases in patients with ischemic or damaged hearts.

PVCs also decrease cardiac output, especially if ectopic beats are frequent or sustained. The decrease in cardiac output with a PVC stems from reduced ventricular diastolic filling time and the loss of atrial kick for that beat. The clinical impact of PVCs hinges on the body's ability to maintain adequate perfusion and the duration of the abnormal rhythm.

To help determine the seriousness of PVCs, ask these questions:
+ *How often do they occur?* In patients with chronic PVCs, an increase in frequency or a change in the pattern of PVCs from the baseline rhythm may signal a more serious condition.
+ *What's the pattern of PVCs?* If the ECG shows a dangerous pattern — such as paired PVCs, PVCs with more than one focus, a bigeminal rhythm, or R-on-T phenomenon (when a PVC strikes on the down slope of the preceding normal T wave) — the patient may require immediate treatment. (See *Patterns of potentially dangerous PVCs,* page 110.)
+ *Are they really PVCs?* Make sure the complex is a PVC, not another, less dangerous arrhythmia. PVCs may be mistaken for ventricular escape beats or

Causes

+ Enhanced automaticity in ventricular conduction system or muscle tissue
+ Electrolyte imbalances
+ Metabolic acidosis
+ Hypoxia
+ Myocardial ischemia or MI
+ Drug intoxication
+ Hypertrophy of ventricular chambers
+ Increased sympathetic stimulation
+ Myocarditis
+ Mitral valve prolapse
+ Caffeine, alcohol, or tobacco use
+ Irritation of ventricles (from pacemaker electrodes)
+ Sympathomimetic drugs

Patterns of potentially dangerous PVCs

Some premature ventricular contractions (PVCs) are more dangerous than others. Here are examples of patterns of potentially dangerous PVCs.

PAIRED PVCS
Two PVCs in a row, called *paired PVCs* or a *ventricular couplet* (see shaded areas), can produce ventricular tachycardia (VT). That's because the second contraction usually meets refractory tissue. A burst, or a *salvo*, of three or more PVCs in a row is considered a run of VT.

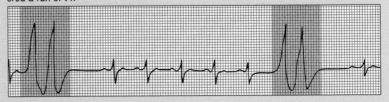

MULTIFORM PVCS
Multiform PVCs, which look different from one another, arise from different sites or from the same site with abnormal conduction (see shaded areas). Multiform PVCs may indicate severe heart disease or digoxin toxicity.

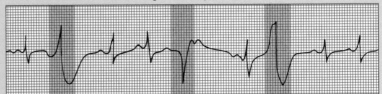

BIGEMINY AND TRIGEMINY
PVCs that occur every other beat *(bigeminy)* or every third beat *(trigeminy)* may indicate increased ventricular irritability, which can result in VT or ventricular fibrillation (see shaded areas). The rhythm strip shown below illustrates ventricular bigeminy.

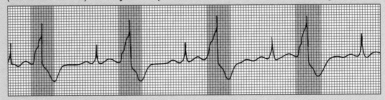

R-ON-T PHENOMENON
In R-on-T phenomenon, a PVC occurs so early that it falls on the T wave of the preceding beat (see shaded area). Because the cells haven't fully repolarized, VT or ventricular fibrillation can result.

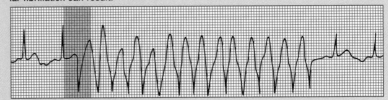

normal impulses with aberrant ventricular conduction. Ventricular escape beats serve as a safety mechanism to protect the heart from ventricular standstill. Some supraventricular impulses may follow an abnormal (aberrant) conduction pathway causing an abnormal appearance to the QRS complex. In any event, never delay treatment if the patient is unstable.

ECG CHARACTERISTICS

Rhythm: Atrial and ventricular rhythms are irregular during PVCs; the underlying rhythm may be regular.

Rate: Atrial and ventricular rates reflect the underlying rhythm.

P wave: Usually absent in the ectopic beat, but with retrograde conduction to the atria, the P wave may appear after the QRS complex. It's usually normal if present in the underlying rhythm.

PR interval: Not measurable except in the underlying rhythm.

QRS complex: Occurrence is earlier than expected. Duration exceeds 0.12 second, with a bizarre and wide configuration. Configuration of the QRS complex is usually normal in the underlying rhythm.

T wave: Occurrence is in opposite direction to QRS complex. When a PVC strikes on the down slope of the preceding normal T wave—the R-on-T phenomenon—it can trigger more serious rhythm disturbances such as ventricular fibrillation.

QT interval: Not usually measured, except in the underlying rhythm.

Other: A PVC may be followed by a compensatory pause, which can be full or incomplete. The sum of a full compensatory pause and the preceding R-R interval is equal to the sum of two R-R intervals of the underlying rhythm. If the sinoatrial (SA) node is depolarized by the PVC, the timing of the SA node is reset, and the compensatory pause is called *incomplete.* In this case, the sum of an incomplete compensatory pause and the preceding R-R interval is less than the sum of two R-R intervals of the underlying rhythm. A PVC occurring between two normally conducted QRS complexes without greatly disturbing the underlying rhythm is referred to as *interpolated.* A full compensatory pause, usually accompanying PVCs, is absent with interpolated PVCs.

Sometimes it's difficult to distinguish PVCs from aberrant ventricular conduction. (See *Distinguishing PVCs from ventricular aberrancy,* pages 112 and 113.)

SIGNS AND SYMPTOMS

The patient experiencing PVCs usually has a normal pulse rate with a momentarily irregular pulse rhythm when a PVC occurs.

With PVCs, the patient will have a weaker pulse wave after the premature beat and a longer-than-normal pause between pulse waves. If the carotid

ECG characteristics
+ *Rhythm*—atrial and ventricular rhythms irregular
+ *Rate*—atrial and ventricular rates reflect underlying rhythm
+ *P wave*—usually absent in ectopic beat
+ *PR interval*—unmeasurable except in underlying rhythm
+ *QRS complex*—duration > 0.12 second, with bizarre, wide configuration
+ *Other*—may be followed by compensatory pause

Signs and symptoms
+ Usually normal pulse rate; however, momentary irregular pulse rhythm when PVC occurs

Distinguishing PVCs from ventricular aberrancy

Perhaps one of the most challenging look-alikes—premature ventricular contractions (PVCs) versus ventricular aberrancy—can sometimes be distinguished with complete confidence only in the electrophysiology laboratory. Ventricular aberrancy, or aberrant ventricular conduction, occurs when an electrical impulse originating in the sinoatrial node, atria, or atrioventricular junction is temporarily conducted abnormally through the bundle branches.

   The abnormal conduction results in a bundle-branch block and usually stems from the arrival of electrical impulses at the bundle branches before the branches have been sufficiently repolarized.

   To distinguish between PVCs and ventricular aberrancy, examine the deflection of the QRS complex in lead V_1. Determine whether the QRS complex is primarily positive or negative. Based on this information, follow these clues to guide your analysis.

MOSTLY POSITIVE QRS

+ Right bundle-branch aberrancy will have a triphasic rSR′ configuration in V_1 and a triphasic qRS configuration in V_6.
+ If there are two positive peaks in V_1 and the left peak is taller, the beat is probably a PVC.
+ PVCs will be monophasic or biphasic in V_1, and biphasic in V_6, with a deep S wave.

COMPARING PVC WITH RIGHT BUNDLE-BRANCH ABERRANCY

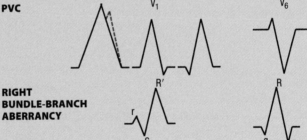

PVC

RIGHT BUNDLE-BRANCH ABERRANCY

Signs and symptoms
(continued)
+ Abnormally early heart sound (when auscultating)
+ May be asymptomatic; palpitations (with frequent PVCs)
+ Hypotension and syncope (decreased cardiac output)

pulse is visible, however, you may see a weaker arterial wave after the premature beat. When auscultating for heart sounds, you'll hear an abnormally early heart sound with each PVC.

   A patient with PVCs may be asymptomatic; however, patients with frequent PVCs may complain of palpitations. The patient may also exhibit signs and symptoms of decreased cardiac output, including hypotension and syncope.

MOSTLY NEGATIVE QRS

✦ Left bundle-branch aberrancy will have a narrow R wave with a quick downstroke in leads V_1 and V_2, with no Q wave in V_6.

✦ PVCs will have a wide R wave (> 0.03 second) and a notched or slurred S-wave downstroke in leads V_1 and V_2, with a duration of > 0.06 second from the onset of the R wave to the deepest point of the S wave in V_1 and V_2, with a Q wave in V_6.

✦ P waves commonly precede aberrancies, but don't generally precede PVCs.

✦ Aberrancies usually have a QRS duration of 0.12 second. PVCs are more likely to have a QRS duration of 0.14 second or more.

COMPARING PVC WITH LEFT BUNDLE-BRANCH ABERRANCY

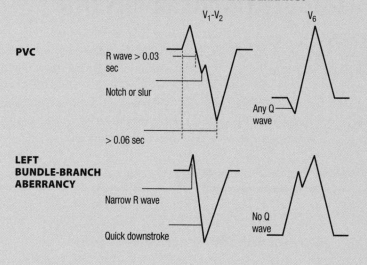

INTERVENTIONS

If the patient is asymptomatic, the arrhythmia probably won't require treatment. If symptoms or a dangerous form of PVCs occur, the type of treatment given will depend on the cause of the problem. Treatment is aimed at cor-

Interventions

✦ Usually unnecessary in asymptomatic patients

✦ If symptoms or dangerous form of PVCs occur, focus on correcting cause

Interventions
(continued)

+ Drugs to suppress ventricular irritability if PVCs have purely cardiac origin
+ Observation of more frequent PVCs in patients with chronic PVCs
+ Continuous ECG monitoring (until effective treatment begins) in patients with PVCs accompanied by serious symptoms

recting the cause. For example, drug therapy may be adjusted or the patient's acidosis corrected.

If PVCs have a purely cardiac origin, drugs to suppress ventricular irritability, such as procainamide, amiodarone, or lidocaine, may be used.

Patients who have recently developed PVCs need prompt assessment, especially if they have underlying heart disease or complex medical problems. Patients with chronic PVCs should be closely observed for the development of more frequent PVCs or more dangerous PVC patterns.

Until effective treatment is begun, patients with PVCs accompanied by serious symptoms should have continuous ECG monitoring and ambulate only with assistance. If the patient is discharged on antiarrhythmic medications, family members should know how to contact the emergency medical system and perform cardiopulmonary resuscitation.

Idioventricular rhythm

+ Originates in escape pacemaker site in ventricles
+ Inherent firing rate usually 20 to 40 beats/minute
+ Acts as safety mechanism by preventing ventricular standstill *(asystole)*
+ Called *AIVR* when rate of ectopic pacemaker site in ventricles is < 100 beats/minute but exceeds inherent ventricular escape rate of 20 to 40 beats/minute

IDIOVENTRICULAR RHYTHM

Idioventricular rhythm, also referred to as *ventricular escape rhythm,* originates in an escape pacemaker site in the ventricles. The inherent firing rate of this ectopic pacemaker is usually 20 to 40 beats/minute. The rhythm acts as a safety mechanism by preventing ventricular standstill, or *asystole*—the absence of electrical activity in the ventricles. When fewer than three QRS complexes arising from the escape pacemaker occur, they're called *ventricular escape beats* or *complexes.* (See *Recognizing idioventricular rhythm.*)

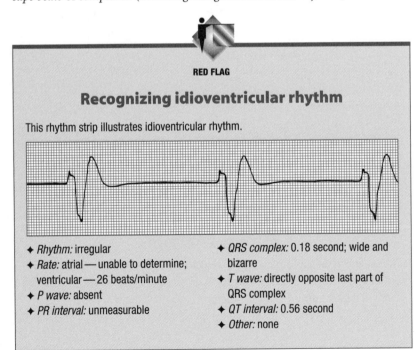

RED FLAG

Recognizing idioventricular rhythm

This rhythm strip illustrates idioventricular rhythm.

+ *Rhythm:* irregular
+ *Rate:* atrial—unable to determine; ventricular—26 beats/minute
+ *P wave:* absent
+ *PR interval:* unmeasurable
+ *QRS complex:* 0.18 second; wide and bizarre
+ *T wave:* directly opposite last part of QRS complex
+ *QT interval:* 0.56 second
+ *Other:* none

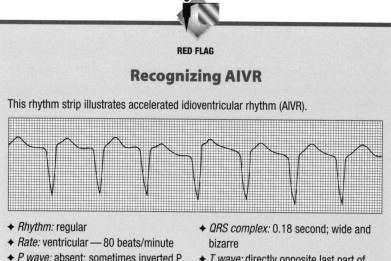

RED FLAG

Recognizing AIVR

This rhythm strip illustrates accelerated idioventricular rhythm (AIVR).

+ *Rhythm:* regular
+ *Rate:* ventricular — 80 beats/minute
+ *P wave:* absent; sometimes inverted P wave follows the QRS complex
+ *PR interval:* unmeasurable

+ *QRS complex:* 0.18 second; wide and bizarre
+ *T wave:* directly opposite last part of QRS complex
+ *QT interval:* usually prolonged
+ *Other:* none

When the rate of an ectopic pacemaker site in the ventricles is under 100 beats/minute but exceeds the inherent ventricular escape rate of 20 to 40 beats/minute, it's called *accelerated idioventricular rhythm (AIVR).* (See *Recognizing AIVR.*) The rate of AIVR isn't fast enough to be considered ventricular tachycardia. The rhythm is usually related to enhanced automaticity of the ventricular tissue. AIVR and idioventricular rhythm share the same ECG characteristics, differing only in heart rate.

CAUSES

Idioventricular rhythms occur when all of the heart's higher pacemakers fail to function or when supraventricular impulses can't reach the ventricles because of a block in the conduction system. Idioventricular rhythms may accompany third-degree heart block. Possible causes of the rhythm include:
+ myocardial ischemia
+ myocardial infarction (MI)
+ digoxin toxicity, beta-adrenergic blockers, calcium antagonists, and tricyclic antidepressants
+ pacemaker failure
+ metabolic imbalances
+ sick sinus syndrome (SSS).

Causes
+ Occurs when higher pacemakers malfunction or when supraventricular impulses can't reach ventricles because of block in conduction system

Other possible causes
+ Myocardial ischemia or MI
+ Digoxin toxicity, beta-adrenergic blockers, calcium antagonists, and tricyclic antidepressants
+ Pacemaker failure
+ Metabolic imbalances
+ SSS

CLINICAL SIGNIFICANCE

Idioventricular rhythm may be transient or continuous. Transient ventricular escape rhythm is usually related to increased parasympathetic effect on the higher pacemaker sites and isn't generally clinically significant. Although idioventricular rhythms act to protect the heart from ventricular standstill, a continuous idioventricular rhythm presents a clinically serious situation.

The slow ventricular rate of this arrhythmia and the associated loss of atrial kick markedly reduce cardiac output. If not rapidly identified and appropriately managed, idioventricular arrhythmias can cause death.

ECG CHARACTERISTICS

Rhythm: Usually, atrial rhythm can't be determined. Ventricular rhythm is usually regular.

Rate: Usually, atrial rate can't be determined. Ventricular rate is 20 to 40 beats/minute.

P wave: Absent.

PR interval: Not measurable because of the absent P wave.

QRS complex: Because of abnormal ventricular depolarization, the QRS complex has a duration longer than 0.12 second, with a wide and bizarre configuration.

T wave: The T wave is abnormal. Deflection usually occurs in the opposite direction from that of the QRS complex.

QT interval: Usually prolonged.

Other: Idioventricular rhythm commonly occurs with third-degree atrioventricular block.

SIGNS AND SYMPTOMS

The patient with continuous idioventricular rhythm is generally symptomatic because of the marked reduction in cardiac output that occurs with the arrhythmia. Blood pressure may be difficult or impossible to auscultate or palpate. The patient may experience dizziness, light-headedness, syncope, or loss of consciousness.

INTERVENTIONS

Treatment should be initiated immediately to increase the patient's heart rate, improve cardiac output, and establish a normal rhythm. Atropine may be administered to increase the heart rate.

If atropine isn't effective or if the patient develops hypotension or other signs of clinical instability, a pacemaker may be needed to reestablish a heart rate that provides enough cardiac output to perfuse organs properly. A tran-

ECG characteristics

+ *Rhythm*—atrial rhythm usually can't be determined; ventricular rhythm usually regular
+ *Rate*—atrial rate usually can't be determined; ventricular rate is 20 to 40 beats/minute
+ *P wave*—absent
+ *PR interval*—unmeasurable
+ *QRS complex*—duration > 0.12 second, with wide, bizarre configuration
+ *T wave*—abnormal; deflection usually occurs in opposite direction from that of QRS complex
+ *QT interval*—usually prolonged

Signs and symptoms

+ Usually symptomatic due to reduction in cardiac output
+ Blood pressure may be difficult to auscultate
+ Possible dizziness, light-headedness, syncope, or loss of consciousness

Interventions

+ Increase patient's heart rate (atropine may be administered), improve cardiac output, and establish normal rhythm
+ Pacemaker (if atropine isn't effective) to reestablish heart rate

scutaneous pacemaker may be used in an emergency until a temporary or transvenous pacemaker can be inserted. (See *Transcutaneous pacemaker*.)

Remember that the goal of treatment doesn't include suppressing the idioventricular rhythm because it acts as a safety mechanism to protect the heart from ventricular standstill. Idioventricular rhythm should never be treated with lidocaine or other antiarrhythmics that would suppress the escape beats.

Patients with idioventricular rhythm need continuous ECG monitoring and constant assessment until treatment restores hemodynamic stability. Keep atropine and pacemaker equipment available at the bedside. Enforce bed rest until an effective heart rate has been maintained and the patient is clinically stable.

Be sure to tell the patient and his family about the serious nature of this arrhythmia and the treatment it requires. If the patient needs a permanent pacemaker, teach the patient and family how it works, how to recognize problems, when to contact the physician, and how pacemaker function will be monitored.

Interventions
(continued)

+ Insert transcutaneous pacemaker (in emergency) until temporary or transvenous is available
+ Don't suppress idioventricular rhythm (for this reason, lidocaine or other antiarrhythmics are contraindicated) as it protects heart from ventricular standstill
+ Monitor ECG and patient until hemodynamic stability is restored

Transcutaneous pacemaker

Transcutaneous pacing, also referred to as *external pacing* or *noninvasive pacing*, involves the delivery of electrical impulses through externally applied cutaneous electrodes. The electrical impulses are conducted through an intact chest wall using skin electrodes placed either in anterior-posterior or sternal-apex positions. (An anterior-posterior placement is shown here.)

Transcutaneous pacing is the initial pacing method of choice in emergency situations because it's the least invasive technique and can be instituted quickly.

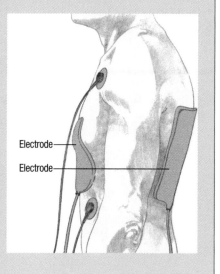

Electrode

Electrode

Ventricular tachycardia

+ Three or more PVCs in a row with ventricular rate > 100 beats/minute
+ May precede ventricular fibrillation and sudden cardiac death
+ Extremely unstable rhythm, which may be sustained (requires immediate treatment) or non-sustained

Causes

+ Enhanced automaticity, reentry within the Purkinje system, or by PVCs occurring during downstroke of preceding T wave
+ Myocardial ischemia or MI
+ CAD
+ Valvular heart disease
+ Heart failure
+ Cardiomyopathy
+ Electrolyte imbalances
+ Drug intoxication

VENTRICULAR TACHYCARDIA

Ventricular tachycardia (VT), also called *V-tach,* occurs when three or more premature ventricular contractions (PVCs) strike in a row and the ventricular rate exceeds 100 beats/minute. This life-threatening arrhythmia may precede ventricular fibrillation and sudden cardiac death.

VT is an extremely unstable rhythm and may be sustained or nonsustained. When it occurs in short, paroxysmal bursts lasting less than 30 seconds and causing few or no symptoms, it's called *non-sustained.* When the rhythm is sustained, however, it requires immediate treatment to prevent death, even in patients initially able to maintain adequate cardiac output. (See *Recognizing VT.*)

CAUSES

This arrhythmia usually results from increased myocardial irritability, which may be triggered by enhanced automaticity, reentry within the Purkinje system, or by PVCs occurring during the downstroke of the preceding T wave.

Other causes of VT include:
+ myocardial ischemia
+ myocardial infarction (MI)
+ coronary artery disease (CAD)
+ valvular heart disease

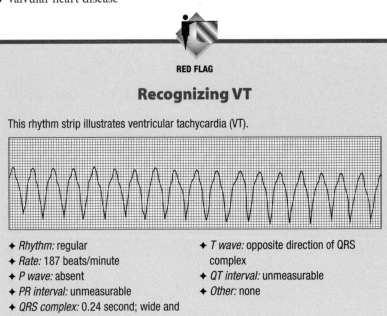

RED FLAG

Recognizing VT

This rhythm strip illustrates ventricular tachycardia (VT).

+ *Rhythm:* regular
+ *Rate:* 187 beats/minute
+ *P wave:* absent
+ *PR interval:* unmeasurable
+ *QRS complex:* 0.24 second; wide and bizarre

+ *T wave:* opposite direction of QRS complex
+ *QT interval:* unmeasurable
+ *Other:* none

✦ heart failure
✦ cardiomyopathy
✦ electrolyte imbalances such as hypokalemia
✦ drug intoxication from digoxin, procainamide, quinidine, or cocaine.

CLINICAL SIGNIFICANCE

VT is significant because of its unpredictability and potential for causing death. A patient may be hemodynamically stable, with a normal pulse and blood pressure; clinically unstable, with hypotension and poor peripheral pulses; or unconscious, without respirations or pulse.

Because of the reduced ventricular filling time and the drop in cardiac output that occurs with this arrhythmia, the patient's condition can quickly deteriorate to ventricular fibrillation (VF) and complete cardiovascular collapse.

ECG CHARACTERISTICS

Rhythm: Atrial rhythm can't be determined. Ventricular rhythm is usually regular but may be slightly irregular.
Rate: Atrial rate can't be determined. Ventricular rate is usually rapid (100 to 250 beats/minute).
P wave: The P wave is usually absent. It may be obscured by the QRS complex; P waves are dissociated from the QRS complexes. Retrograde P waves may be present.
PR interval: Not measurable because the P wave can't be seen in most cases.
QRS complex: Duration is greater than 0.12 second; it usually has a bizarre appearance with increased amplitude. QRS complexes in monomorphic VT have a uniform shape. In polymorphic VT, the shape of the QRS complex constantly changes.
T wave: If the T wave is visible, it occurs in the opposite direction of the QRS complex.
QT interval: Not measurable.
Other: Ventricular flutter and torsades de pointes are two variations of this arrhythmia. *Torsades de pointes i*s a special variation of polymorphic VT. (See *Recognizing torsades de pointes,* page 120.) Although a relatively rare occurrence, torsades de pointes is sometimes difficult to distinguish from ventricular flutter. (See *Distinguishing ventricular flutter from torsades de pointes,* page 121.)

Sometimes distinguishing VT from supraventricular tachycardia (SVT) can be extremely challenging, especially in the setting of aberrant ventricular conduction. (See *Distinguishing VT from SVT,* pages 122 and 123.)

ECG characteristics

✦ *Rhythm*—atrial rhythm can't be determined; ventricular rhythm usually regular (but may be slightly irregular)
✦ *Rate*—atrial rate can't be determined; ventricular rate usually rapid (100 to 250 beats/minute)
✦ *P wave*—usually absent
✦ *PR interval*—unmeasurable
✦ *QRS complex*—duration is > 0.12 second; usually has bizarre appearance (with increased amplitude)
✦ *T wave*—if visible, occurs in opposite direction of QRS complex
✦ *Other*—ventricular flutter and torsades de pointes (special variation of polymorphic VT)

Recognizing torsades de pointes

Characteristics of torsades de pointes *(twisting of points)*:

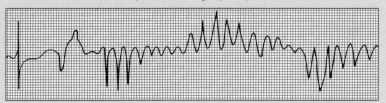

◆ *Rhythm:* atrial rhythm—can't be determined; ventricular rhythm—regular or irregular
◆ *Rate:* atrial rate—can't be determined; ventricular rate—150 to 250 beats/minute
◆ *P wave:* not identifiable because it's buried in the QRS complex
◆ *PR interval:* not applicable because P wave can't be identified

◆ *QRS complex:* usually wide with a phasic variation in its electrical polarity, shown by complexes that point downward for several beats, and vice versa
◆ *T wave:* not discernible
◆ *QT interval:* prolonged
◆ *Other:* may be paroxysmal, starting and stopping suddenly

Signs and symptoms
◆ May be minor initially (still requires rapid intervention)
◆ Weak or absent pulses (common)
◆ Hypotension and decreased LOC, quickly leading to unresponsiveness if left untreated

Interventions
◆ With pulseless VT, treatment is the same as that for VF (immediate defibrillation)
◆ With detectable pulse, treatment depends on whether the patient is *unstable* or *stable*

SIGNS AND SYMPTOMS

Although some patients have only minor symptoms initially, they still require rapid intervention to prevent cardiovascular collapse. Most patients with VT have weak or absent pulses. Low cardiac output will cause hypotension and a decreased level of consciousness (LOC), quickly leading to unresponsiveness if left untreated. VT may prompt angina, heart failure, or a substantial decrease in organ perfusion.

INTERVENTIONS

Treatment depends on the patient's clinical status. Is the patient conscious? Does the patient have spontaneous respirations? Is a palpable carotid pulse present?

Patients with pulseless VT are treated the same as those with VF and require immediate defibrillation. Treatment for patients with a detectable pulse depends on whether they're unstable or stable.

Unstable patients generally have ventricular rates greater than 150 beats/minute and have serious signs and symptoms related to the tachycardia,

LOOK-ALIKES

Distinguishing ventricular flutter from torsades de pointes

Torsades de pointes is a variant form of ventricular tachycardia, with a rapid ventricular rate that varies between 250 and 350 beats/minute. It's characterized by QRS complexes that gradually change back and forth, with the amplitude of each successive complex gradually increasing and decreasing. This results in an overall outline of the rhythm commonly described as *spindle-shaped*.

Ventricular flutter, although rarely recognized, results from the rapid, regular, repetitive beating of the ventricles. It's produced by a single ventricular focus firing at a rapid rate of 250 to 350 beats/minute. The hallmark of this arrhythmia is its smooth sine-wave appearance.

The illustrations shown here highlight key differences in the two arrhythmias.

VENTRICULAR FLUTTER
✦ Smooth, sine-wave appearance

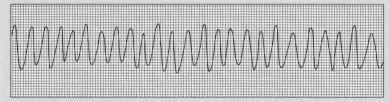

TORSADES DE POINTES
✦ Spindle-shaped appearance

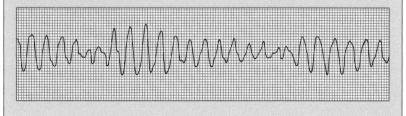

which may include hypotension, shortness of breath, chest pain, or altered LOC. These patients are usually treated with immediate synchronized cardioversion.

A clinically stable patient with wide-complex VT and no signs of heart failure is treated differently. Treatment for these patients is determined by

Interventions
(continued)

Unstable
✦ Ventricular rates > 150 beats/ minute with serious signs and symptoms
✦ Immediate synchronized cardioversion

Stable
✦ Treatment for patients with wide-complex VT and no signs of heart failure is different

Distinguishing VT from SVT

Differentiating ventricular tachycardia (VT) from supraventricular tachycardia (SVT) with aberrancy is difficult. Careful assessment of a 12-lead ECG or rhythm strip can help you differentiate the arrhythmia with 90% accuracy.

Begin by looking at the deflection — negative or positive. Then use these illustrations to guide your assessment. If the QRS complex is wide and mostly negative in deflection in V_1 or MCL_1, use these clues.

VENTRICULAR TACHYCARDIA

✦ If the QRS complex has an R wave $\geq$ 0.04 second, a slurred S (shown below, shaded), or a notched S (shown at right) on the downstroke, suspect VT.

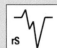

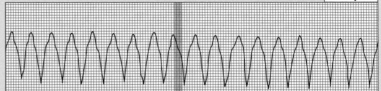

SUPRAVENTRICULAR TACHYCARDIA

✦ If the QRS complex has an R wave $\leq$ 0.04 second and a swift, straight S on the downstroke (shown below, shaded, and at right), suspect SVT with aberrancy.

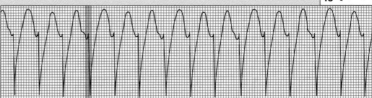

If the QRS complex is wide and mostly positive in deflection in V_1 or MCL_1, use these clues.

VENTRICULAR TACHYCARDIA

✦ If the QRS complex is biphasic, suspect VT.

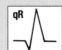
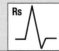

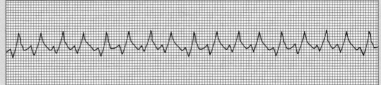

Distinguishing VT from SVT *(continued)*

SUPRAVENTRICULAR TACHYCARDIA

◆ If the beat is triphasic, similar to a right bundle-branch block, suspect SVT with aberrancy.

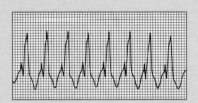

rR′

triphasic rSR′

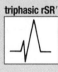

Here are additional clues you can use if the QRS complex is wide and mostly positive in deflection in lead V_1 or MCL_1.

If the QRS complex is tall and shaped like rabbit ears, with the left peak taller than the right, suspect VT.	If the QRS complex is monophasic, suspect VT.	If you still have difficulty differentiating the rhythm, look at V_6 or MCL_6. If the S wave is larger than the R wave, suspect VT.	If any Q wave is present, suspect VT.

Taller left peak

QRS

rS

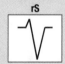

Q

Other general criteria can also help you differentiate VT from SVT with aberrancy.

◆ A QRS complex > 0.14 second suggests VT.
◆ A regular, wide, complex rhythm suggests VT.
◆ An irregular, wide, complex rhythm suggests SVT with aberrancy.
◆ Concordant V leads (the QRS complex either mainly positive or mainly negative in all V leads) suggest VT.
◆ Atrioventricular dissociation suggests VT.

Interventions
(continued)

Stable

◆ Depends on whether VT is monomorphic or polymorphic, whether cardiac function is normal or impaired, and whether baseline QT interval is normal or prolonged

whether the VT is monomorphic or polymorphic, whether the patient has normal or impaired cardiac function, and whether the baseline QT interval is normal or prolonged. (See *Stable monomorphic or polymorphic ventricular tachycardia algorithm,* page 124.)

Stable monomorphic or polymorphic ventricular tachycardia algorithm

Cardioversion is an appropriate, immediate treatment for any stable ventricular tachycardia (VT). Alternatives to this treatment depend on the type of VT, the patient's cardiac function, and the configuration of the QT interval. In monomorphic VT, QRS complexes keep the same form or appearance. In polymorphic VT, QRS complexes occur in more than one form, varying in appearance.

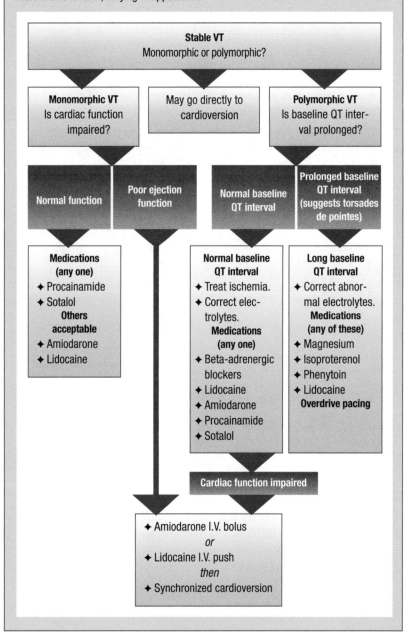

Patients with chronic, recurrent episodes of VT unresponsive to drug therapy may need an implanted cardioverter-defibrillator (ICD). This device is a permanent solution to recurrent episodes of VT. (See *Understanding the ICD*.)

A 12-lead ECG and all other available clinical information is critical for establishing a specific diagnosis in a stable patient with wide QRS complex tachycardia of unknown type. If a definitive diagnosis of SVT or VT can't be established, the patient's treatment should be guided by whether cardiac function is preserved (ejection fraction greater than 40%).

Be sure to teach patients and families about the serious nature of this arrhythmia and the need for prompt treatment. If your stable patient is undergoing electrical cardioversion, inform him that he'll be given a sedative, and possibly an analgesic, prior to the procedure.

If a patient will be discharged with an ICD or a prescription for long-term antiarrhythmics, make sure that family members know how to use the emergency medical system and how to perform cardiopulmonary resuscitation.

 AGE CHANGE Torsades de pointes at an early age is usually caused by congenital long QT syndrome. Ask the parents about a family history of sudden cardiac death or sudden infant death syndrome.

Interventions
(continued)
Stable
+ Implanted ICD for chronic, recurrent episodes of VT unresponsive to drug therapy
+ Should be guided by whether cardiac function is preserved (ejection fraction > 40%) if definitive diagnoses of SVT or VT can't be made

---

Understanding the ICD

The implantable cardioverter-defibrillator (ICD) has a programmable pulse generator and lead system that monitors the heart's activity, detects ventricular arrhythmias and other tachyarrhythmias, and responds with appropriate therapies. The range of therapies includes antitachycardia and antibradycardia pacing, cardioversion, and defibrillation. Newer defibrillators can also pace the atrium and the ventricle.

Implantation of the ICD is similar to that of a permanent pacemaker. The cardiologist positions the lead (or leads) transvenously in the endocardium of the right ventricle (and the right atrium, if both chambers require pacing). The lead connects to a generator box implanted in the right or left upper chest near the clavicle.

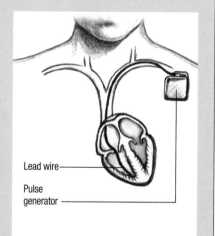

Lead wire

Pulse generator

Ventricular fibrillation

+ Chaotic, disorganized pattern of electrical activity
+ Arises from electrical impulses coming from multiple ectopic pacemakers in ventricles
+ Produces no effective ventricular activity or contractions and no cardiac output
+ Most common cause of sudden cardiac death if left untreated

Causes

+ CAD
+ Myocardial ischemia or MI
+ Underlying VT
+ Underlying heart disease
+ Acid-base imbalance
+ Electric shock
+ Severe hypothermia
+ Drug toxicity
+ Electrolyte imbalances

VENTRICULAR FIBRILLATION

Ventricular fibrillation, commonly called *V-fib* or *VF*, is characterized by a chaotic, disorganized pattern of electrical activity. The pattern arises from electrical impulses coming from multiple ectopic pacemakers in the ventricles.

The arrhythmia produces no effective ventricular mechanical activity or contractions and no cardiac output. Untreated VF is the most common cause of sudden cardiac death in people outside of a health care facility. (See *Recognizing VF*.)

CAUSES

Causes of VF include:

+ coronary artery disease (CAD)
+ myocardial ischemia
+ myocardial infarction (MI)

RED FLAG

Recognizing VF

Characteristics of ventricular fibrillation (VF):

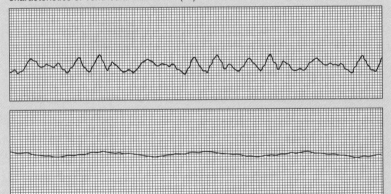

+ *Rhythm:* chaotic
+ *Rate:* can't be determined
+ *P wave:* absent
+ *PR interval:* unmeasurable
+ *QRS complex:* indiscernible
+ *T wave:* indiscernible
+ *QT interval:* not applicable

+ *Other:* the presence of large fibrillatory waves indicates coarse VF (as shown in the first ECG strip, top); the presence of small fibrillatory waves indicates fine VF (as shown in the second ECG strip, bottom)

+ untreated ventricular tachycardia (VT)
+ underlying heart disease such as dilated cardiomyopathy
+ acid-base imbalance
+ electric shock
+ severe hypothermia
+ drug toxicity, including digoxin, quinidine, and procainamide
+ electrolyte imbalances, such as hypokalemia, hyperkalemia, and hypercalcemia.

CLINICAL SIGNIFICANCE

With VF, the ventricular muscle quivers, replacing effective muscular contraction with completely ineffective contraction. Cardiac output falls to zero and, if allowed to continue, leads to ventricular standstill and death.

ECG CHARACTERISTICS

Rhythm: Atrial rhythm can't be determined. Ventricular rhythm has no pattern or regularity. Ventricular electrical activity appears as fibrillatory waves with no recognizable pattern.
Rate: Atrial and ventricular rates can't be determined.
P wave: Can't be determined.
PR interval: Can't be determined.
QRS complex: Duration can't be determined.
T wave: Can't be determined.
QT interval: Not applicable.
Other: Coarse fibrillatory waves are generally associated with greater chances of successful electrical defibrillation than smaller amplitude waves. Fibrillatory waves become finer as hypoxemia and acidosis progress, making the VF more resistant to defibrillation.

SIGNS AND SYMPTOMS

The patient in VF is in full cardiac arrest, unresponsive, and without a detectable blood pressure or central pulses. Whenever you see an ECG pattern resembling VF, check the patient immediately and initiate definitive treatment.

INTERVENTIONS

When faced with a rhythm that appears to be VF, always assess the patient first. Other events can mimic VF on an ECG strip, including interference from an electric razor, shivering, or seizure activity.

Immediate defibrillation is the most effective treatment for VF. Cardiopulmonary resuscitation (CPR) must be performed until the defibrillator

ECG characteristics
+ *Rhythm*—atrial rhythm can't be determined; ventricular rhythm has no pattern or regularity
+ *Rate*—atrial and ventricular rates can't be determined
+ *P wave*—can't be determined
+ *PR interval*—can't be determined
+ *QRS complex*—duration can't be determined
+ *T wave*—can't be determined
+ *Other*—coarse fibrillatory waves associated with greater chance for successful defibrillation

Signs and symptoms
+ Unresponsive with no detectable blood pressure or central pulses

Interventions
+ Assess patient immediately when faced with VF rhythm
+ Immediate defibrillation is most effective
+ CPR until defibrillator arrives, preserving oxygen supply to vital organs

Interventions
(continued)

+ Drugs (epinephrine, vasopressin) for persistent VF if initial three attempts at electrical defibrillation fail
+ Antiarrhythmics (amiodarone, magnesium)
+ Defibrillation to encourage SA node to resume control of heart's electrical activity
+ AEDs to provide early defibrillation (especially in out-of-hospital settings); family members may need instruction

arrives to preserve oxygen supply to the brain and other vital organs. Drugs such as epinephrine and vasopressin may be used for persistent VF if the initial three attempts at electrical defibrillation fail to correct the arrhythmia. Antiarrhythmic agents, such as amiodarone and magnesium, may also be considered. (See *VF and pulseless VT algorithm.*)

In defibrillation, two electrode pads are applied to the chest wall. Current is then directed through the pads and, subsequently, the patient's chest and heart. The current causes the myocardium to completely depolarize, which, in turn, encourages the sinoatrial node to resume normal control of the heart's electrical activity.

One electrode pad is placed to the right of the upper sternum, and one is placed over the fifth or sixth intercostal space at the left anterior axillary line. During cardiac surgery, internal paddles are placed directly on the myocardium.

Automated external defibrillators (AEDs) are increasingly being used, especially in the out-of-hospital setting, to provide early defibrillation. After a patient is confirmed to be unresponsive, breathless, and pulseless, the AED power is turned on and the electrode pads and cables attached. The AED can analyze the patient's cardiac rhythm and provide the caregiver with step-by-step instructions on how to proceed. These defibrillators can be used by people without medical experience as long as they're trained in the proper use of the device. (See *Understanding the AED.*)

For the patient in VF, successful resuscitation requires rapid recognition of the problem and prompt defibrillation. Many health care facilities and emergency medical systems have established protocols so that health care workers can initiate prompt treatment. Make sure you know the location of your facility's emergency equipment, and that you know how to use it.

Understanding the AED

Automated external defibrillators (AEDs) vary with the manufacturer, but the basic components of each device are similar. This illustration shows a typical AED and how to place electrodes properly.

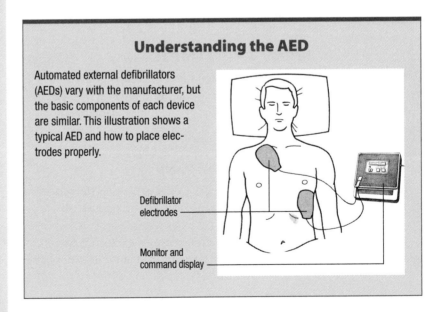

Defibrillator electrodes

Monitor and command display

VF and pulseless VT algorithm

Ventricular fibrillation (VF) and pulseless ventricular tachycardia (VT) require aggressive, systematic treatment. Follow this algorithm for patients with these arrhythmias.

Primary ABCD survey

Focus: basic cardiopulmonary resuscitation and defibrillation

- Check responsiveness.
- Activate emergency response system.
- Call for defibrillator.
- **A** Airway: Open the airway.
- **B** Breathing: Provide positive-pressure ventilations.
- **C** Circulation: Give chest compressions.
- **D** Defibrillation: Assess for VF or pulseless VT and defibrillate up to three times (200 joules, 200 to 300 joules, 360 joules, or equivalent biphasic), if necessary.

Rhythm after first three defibrillations?

Persistent or recurrent VF or VT

Secondary ABCD survey

Focus: more advanced assessments and treatments

- **A** Airway: Insert airway device as soon as possible.
- **B** Breathing: Confirm airway device placement by examination plus confirmation device.
- **B** Breathing: Secure airway device: purpose-made tube holders preferred.
- **B** Breathing: Confirm effective oxygenation and ventilation.
- **C** Circulation: Establish I.V. access.
- **C** Circulation: Identify rhythm and monitor.
- **C** Circulation: Administer drugs appropriate for rhythm and condition.
- **D** Differential diagnosis: Search for and treat identified reversible causes.

- Epinephrine I.V. push; repeat every 3 to 5 minutes

or

- Vasopressin I.V.; single dose, one time only

Resume attempts to defibrillate.
1 × 360 joules (or equivalent biphasic) within 30 to 60 seconds

Consider antiarrhythmics and buffers.

- Amiodarone
- Lidocaine
- Magnesium
- Procainamide
- Sodium bicarbonate

Resume attempts to defibrillate.

You'll also need to teach the patient and family how to use the emergency medical system following discharge from the facility. Family members may need instruction in CPR and in how to use the AED. Teach them about long-term therapies that help prevent recurrent episodes of VF, including anti-arrhythmic drug therapy and implantable cardioverter-defibrillators.

Asystole

+ Absence of discernible electrical activity in ventricles (also called *ventricular standstill*)
+ Impulses aren't conducted to ventricles, but some electrical activity may be evident in atria
+ Results from prolonged period of cardiac arrest without effective resuscitation
+ Must be distinguished from fine VF and confirmed in more than one ECG lead

Causes

+ Hypovolemia
+ MI
+ Severe electrolyte disturbances
+ Massive pulmonary embolism
+ Hypoxia
+ Severe, uncorrected acid-base disturbances
+ Drug overdose
+ Hypothermia
+ Cardiac tamponade
+ Tension pneumothorax

ASYSTOLE

Ventricular asystole, also called *asystole* and *ventricular standstill,* is the absence of discernible electrical activity in the ventricles. Although some electrical activity may be evident in the atria, these impulses aren't conducted to the ventricles. (See *Recognizing asystole.*)

Asystole usually results from a prolonged period of cardiac arrest without effective resuscitation. It's important to distinguish asystole from fine ventricular fibrillation, which is managed differently. Therefore, asystole must be confirmed in more than one ECG lead.

CAUSES

Possible reversible causes of asystole include:

+ hypovolemia
+ myocardial infarction (MI) (coronary thrombosis)
+ severe electrolyte disturbances, especially hyperkalemia and hypokalemia
+ massive pulmonary embolism
+ hypoxia
+ severe, uncorrected acid-base disturbances, especially metabolic acidosis
+ drug overdose
+ hypothermia
+ cardiac tamponade
+ tension pneumothorax.

CLINICAL SIGNIFICANCE

Without ventricular electrical activity, ventricular contractions can't occur. As a result, cardiac output drops to zero and vital organs are no longer perfused. Asystole has been called the *arrhythmia of death* and is typically considered to be a confirmation of death, rather than an arrhythmia to be treated.

The patient with asystole is completely unresponsive, without spontaneous respirations or pulse (cardiopulmonary arrest). Without immediate initiation of cardiopulmonary resuscitation (CPR) and rapid identification and treatment of the underlying cause, the condition quickly becomes irreversible.

RED FLAG

Recognizing asystole

Characteristics of asystole:

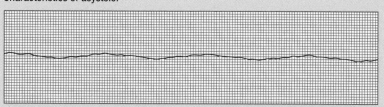

- ✦ *Rhythm:* atrial rhythm—usually indiscernible; no ventricular rhythm
- ✦ *Rate:* atrial rate—usually indiscernible; no ventricular rate
- ✦ *P wave:* may be present
- ✦ *PR interval:* unmeasurable
- ✦ *QRS complex:* absent, or occasional escape beats
- ✦ *T wave:* absent
- ✦ *QT interval:* unmeasurable
- ✦ *Other:* absence of electrical activity in the ventricles results in a nearly flat line

ECG CHARACTERISTICS

Rhythm: Atrial rhythm is usually indiscernible; no ventricular rhythm is present.

Rate: Atrial rate is usually indiscernible; no ventricular rate is present.

P wave: May be present.

PR interval: Not measurable.

QRS complex: Absent or occasional escape beats.

T wave: Absent.

QT interval: Not measurable.

Other: On a rhythm strip, asystole looks like a nearly flat line (except for changes caused by chest compressions during CPR). In a patient with a pacemaker, pacer spikes may be evident on the strip but no P wave or QRS complex occurs in response to the stimulus.

SIGNS AND SYMPTOMS

The patient will be unresponsive and have no spontaneous respirations, discernible pulse, or blood pressure.

INTERVENTIONS

Immediate treatment for asystole includes effective CPR, supplemental oxygen, and advanced airway control with tracheal intubation. Resuscitation should be attempted unless evidence exists that these efforts shouldn't be ini-

ECG characteristics
- ✦ *Rhythm*—atrial rhythm usually indiscernible; no ventricular rhythm present
- ✦ *Rate*—atrial rate usually indiscernible; no ventricular rate present
- ✦ *P wave*—possibly present
- ✦ *PR interval*—unmeasurable
- ✦ *QRS complex*—absent or occasional escape beats
- ✦ *T wave*—absent
- ✦ *QT interval*—unmeasurable
- ✦ *Other*—looks like nearly flat line on rhythm strip

Signs and symptoms
- ✦ Unresponsive, with no spontaneous respirations, discernible pulse, or blood pressure

Interventions
- ✦ Effective CPR, supplemental oxygen, and advanced airway control with tracheal intubation

Interventions
(continued)

+ Check more than one lead to verify asystole
+ Treat potentially reversible causes first
+ Early transcutaneous pacing
+ I.V. epinephrine and atropine, as ordered

tiated, such as when a do-not-resuscitate order is in effect. (See *Asystole algorithm.*)

Remember to verify the presence of asystole by checking more than one ECG lead. Priority must also be given to searching for and treating identified potentially reversible causes, such as hypovolemia, cardiac tamponade, and tension pneumothorax. Early transcutaneous pacing may be considered, and I.V. epinephrine and atropine is administered, as ordered.

Be aware that pulseless electrical activity (PEA) can appear as any cardiac rhythm, including asystole. Know how to recognize this problem and treat it. (See *Pulseless electrical activity.*)

With persistent asystole (despite appropriate management), consider terminating resuscitation.

Facts about pulseless electrical activity

+ Characterized by some type of electrical activity, but no detectable pulse
+ Organized electrical depolarization occurs, but no synchronous shortening of myocardial fibers

Causes
+ Hypovolemia, hypoxia, tension pneumothorax, cardiac tamponade, massive pulmonary embolism, hypothermia, hyperkalemia and hypokalemia, massive acute MI, and drug overdoses

Treatment
+ Rapid identification and treatment of underlying reversible causes
+ CPR, tracheal intubation, and I.V. epinephrine or atropine

RED FLAG

Pulseless electrical activity

Pulseless electrical activity (PEA) defines a group of arrhythmias characterized by the presence of some type of electrical activity without a detectable pulse. Although organized electrical depolarization occurs, no synchronous shortening of the myocardial fibers occurs. As a result, no mechanical activity or contractions take place.

CAUSES
The most common causes of PEA include hypovolemia, hypoxia, acidosis, tension pneumothorax, cardiac tamponade, massive pulmonary embolism, hypothermia, hyperkalemia and hypokalemia, massive acute myocardial infarction, and overdoses of drugs such as tricyclic antidepressants.

TREATMENT
Rapid identification and treatment of underlying reversible causes is critical for treating PEA. For example, hypovolemia is treated with volume expansion. Tension pneumothorax is treated with needle decompression.

Institute cardiopulmonary resuscitation, tracheal intubation, and I.V. administration of epinephrine or atropine.

Asystole algorithm

Few patients with asystole survive. The treatment goal is to reestablish a heart rhythm. Treatment includes pacing and appropriate medications to stimulate impulse conduction. Use this algorithm to guide treatment of the patient with asystole.

Primary ABCD survey
Focus: basic cardiopulmonary resuscitation and defibrillation

+ Check responsiveness.
+ Activate emergency response system.
+ Call for defibrillator.
+ **A** Airway: Open the airway.
+ **B** Breathing: Provide positive-pressure ventilations.
+ **C** Circulation: Give chest compressions.

+ **C** Circulation: Confirm true asystole.
+ **D** Defibrillation: Assess for ventricular fibrillation (VF) or pulseless ventricular tachycardia (VT); defibrillate, if indicated.
+ Rapid scene survey: Any evidence personnel should not attempt resuscitation?

Secondary ABCD survey
Focus: more advanced assessments and treatments

+ **A** Airway: Place airway device as soon as possible.
+ **B** Breathing: Confirm airway device placement by examination plus confirmation device.
+ **B** Breathing: Secure airway device: purpose-made tube holders preferred.
+ **B** Breathing: Confirm effective oxygenation and ventilation.

+ **C** Circulation: Confirm true asystole.
+ **C** Circulation: Establish I.V. access.
+ **C** Circulation: Identify rhythm on monitor.
+ **C** Circulation: Give medications appropriate for rhythm and condition.
+ **D** Differential diagnosis: Search for and treat identified reversible causes.

Transcutaneous pacing
If considered, perform immediately.

Epinephrine I.V. push; repeat every 3 to 5 minutes.

Atropine I.V. push

Asystole persists
Withhold or cease resuscitation efforts?

+ Consider quality of resuscitation?
+ Atypical clinical features present?
+ Support for cease-efforts protocols in place?

Atrioventricular blocks

Atrioventricular (AV) heart block refers to an interruption or delay in the conduction of electrical impulses between the atria and the ventricles. The block can occur at the AV node, the bundle of His, or the bundle branches. When the site of the block is the bundle of His or the bundle branches, the block is referred to as *infranodal AV block*. AV block can be partial (first or second degree) or complete (third degree).

The heart's electrical impulses normally originate in the sinoatrial node, so when those impulses are blocked at the AV node, atrial rates are usually normal (60 to 100 beats/minute). The clinical significance of the block depends on the number of impulses completely blocked and the resulting ventricular rate. A slow ventricular rate can decrease cardiac output and cause symptoms such as light-headedness, hypotension, and confusion.

CAUSES OF ATRIOVENTRICULAR BLOCK

A variety of factors may lead to AV block, including underlying heart conditions, use of certain drugs, congenital anomalies, and conditions that disrupt the cardiac conduction system.

Typical causes of AV block include:

✦ myocardial ischemia, which impairs cellular function so that cells repolarize more slowly or incompletely. The injured cells, in turn, may conduct im-

Causes

+ Myocardial ischemia
+ MI
+ Excessive serum levels of, or exaggerated response to drug
+ Lesions along conduction pathway
+ Congenital anomalies
+ Inadvertent damage to heart's conduction system during cardiac surgery
+ Radiofrequency ablation

pulses slowly or inconsistently. Relief of the ischemia may restore normal function to the AV node.

+ myocardial infarction (MI), in which cellular necrosis or death occurs. If the necrotic cells are part of the conduction system, they may no longer conduct impulses and a permanent AV block occurs.

+ excessive serum levels of, or an exaggerated response to a drug. This response can cause AV block or increase the likelihood that a block will develop. The drugs may increase the refractory period of a portion of the conduction system. Although many antiarrhythmics can have this effect, the drugs more commonly known to cause or exacerbate AV blocks include digoxin, amiodarone, beta-adrenergic blockers, and calcium channel blockers.

+ lesions, including calcium and fibrotic, along the conduction pathway.

+ congenital anomalies such as congenital ventricular septal defects that involve cardiac structures and affect the conduction system. Anomalies of the conduction system, such as an AV node that doesn't conduct impulses, can also occur in the absence of structural defects.

AV block can also be caused by inadvertent damage to the heart's conduction system during surgery. Damage is most likely to occur in operations involving the aortic, mitral, or tricuspid valve or in the closure of a ventricular septal defect. If the injury involves tissues adjacent to the surgical site and the conduction system isn't physically disrupted, the block may be temporary. If a portion of the conduction system is severed, permanent block results.

Similar disruption of the conduction system can occur from a procedure called *radiofrequency ablation*. In this invasive procedure, a transvenous catheter is used to locate the area in the heart that participates in initiating or perpetuating certain tachyarrhythmias. Radiofrequency energy is then delivered to the myocardium through this catheter to produce a small area of necrosis at that spot. The damaged tissue can no longer cause or participate in the tachyarrhythmia. If the energy is delivered close to the AV node, bundle of His, or bundle branches, however, AV block can result and the patient may need a permanent pacemaker.

Classification

+ Classified according to site of block and severity of conduction abnormality
+ Severity classified as first degree; second degree, type I (Wenckebach, Mobitz I); second degree, type II (Mobitz II); and third degree (complete)

CLASSIFICATION OF ATRIOVENTRICULAR BLOCK

Atrioventricular (AV) blocks are classified according to the site of block and the severity of the conduction abnormality. The sites of AV block include the AV node, bundle of His, and bundle branches.

Severity of AV block is classified in degrees: first-degree AV block; second-degree AV block, type I (Wenckebach or Mobitz I); second-degree AV block, type II (Mobitz II) AV block; and third-degree (complete) AV block. The classification system for AV blocks aids in the determination of the patient's treatment and prognosis.

FIRST-DEGREE ATRIOVENTRICULAR BLOCK

First-degree atrioventricular (AV) block occurs when there's a delay in the conduction of electrical impulses from the atria to the ventricles. This delay usually occurs at the level of the AV node, or bundle of His. First-degree AV block is characterized by a PR interval greater than 0.20 second. This interval remains constant beat to beat. Electrical impulses are conducted through the normal conduction pathway. However, conduction of these impulses takes longer than normal.

CAUSES

First-degree AV block may result from myocardial ischemia or myocardial infarction (MI), myocarditis, or degenerative changes in the heart associated with aging. The condition may also be caused by drugs, such as digoxin, calcium channel blockers, and beta-adrenergic blockers.

CLINICAL SIGNIFICANCE

First-degree AV block may cause no symptoms in a healthy person. The arrhythmia may be transient, especially if it occurs secondary to drugs or ischemia early in the course of an MI. The presence of first-degree block, the least dangerous type of AV block, indicates a delay in the conduction of electrical impulses through the normal conduction pathway. In general, a rhythm strip with this block looks like normal sinus rhythm except that the PR interval is longer than normal.

Because first-degree AV block can progress to a more severe type of AV block, the patient's cardiac rhythm should be monitored for changes. (See *Recognizing first-degree AV block,* page 138.)

ECG CHARACTERISTICS

Rhythm: Atrial and ventricular rhythms are regular.
Rate: Atrial and ventricular rates are the same and within normal limits.
P wave: Normal size and configuration; each P wave followed by a QRS complex.
PR interval: Prolonged (greater than 0.20 second) but constant.
QRS complex: Duration usually remains within normal limits if the conduction delay occurs in the AV node. If the QRS duration exceeds 0.12 second, the conduction delay may be in the His-Purkinje system.
T wave: Normal size and configuration unless the QRS complex is prolonged.
QT interval: Usually within normal limits.
Other: None.

First-degree AV block
+ Delayed conduction of electrical impulses from atria to ventricles
+ PR interval > 0.20 second (remains constant beat to beat)

Causes
+ Myocardial ischemia or MI
+ Myocarditis
+ Degenerative heart changes (aging)
+ Certain drugs

ECG characteristics
+ *Rhythm* — atrial and ventricular rhythms regular
+ *Rate* — atrial and ventricular rates same and within normal limits
+ *P wave* — normal size and configuration; followed by a QRS complex
+ *PR interval* — prolonged (> 0.20 second), but constant
+ *QRS complex* — duration usually remaining within normal limits

Recognizing first-degree AV block

This rhythm strip illustrates first-degree atrioventricular (AV) block.

+ *Rhythm:* regular
+ *Rate:* 75 beats/minute
+ *P wave:* normal
+ *PR interval:* 0.32 second; > 0.20 second (see shaded area)
+ *QRS complex:* 0.08 second
+ *T wave:* normal
+ *QT interval:* 0.40 second
+ *Other:* PR interval — prolonged but constant

Signs and symptoms

+ Pulse rate usually normal; rhythm regular
+ Usually asymptomatic; but, with long PR interval, longer interval between S_1 and S_2

Interventions

+ Identify and correct underlying cause (such as if drug is cause, dosage may be reduced or discontinued)
+ Monitor ECG to detect progression to more serious form of block

SIGNS AND SYMPTOMS

The patient's pulse rate will usually be normal and the rhythm will be regular. Most patients with first-degree AV block are asymptomatic because cardiac output isn't significantly affected. If the PR interval is extremely long, a longer interval between S_1 and S_2 may be noted on cardiac auscultation.

INTERVENTIONS

Treatment generally focuses on identification and correction of the underlying cause. For example, if a drug is causing the AV block, the dosage may be reduced or the drug discontinued. Close monitoring can help detect progression of first-degree AV block to a more serious form of block.

Evaluate a patient with first-degree AV block for underlying causes that can be corrected, such as drugs or myocardial ischemia. Observe the ECG for progression of the block to a more severe form. Administer digoxin, calcium channel blockers, and beta-adrenergic blockers cautiously.

Second-degree AV block

+ Some electrical impulses from AV node are blocked and some are conducted normally
+ Subdivided into type I and type II

SECOND-DEGREE ATRIOVENTRICULAR BLOCK

Second-degree atrioventricular (AV) block occurs when some of the electrical impulses from the AV node are blocked and some are conducted through normal conduction pathways. Second-degree AV block is subdivided into type I second-degree AV block and type II second-degree AV block.

TYPE I SECOND-DEGREE AV BLOCK

Also called *Wenckebach* or *Mobitz I block,* type I second-degree AV block occurs when each successive impulse from the sinoatrial (SA) node is delayed slightly longer than the previous impulse. (See *Recognizing type I second-degree AV block.*) This pattern of progressive prolongation of the PR interval continues until an impulse fails to be conducted to the ventricles.

Usually only a single impulse is blocked from reaching the ventricles, and following this nonconducted P wave or dropped beat, the pattern is repeated. This repetitive sequence of two or more consecutive beats followed by a dropped beat results in "group beating." Type I second-degree AV block generally occurs at the level of the AV node.

Causes

Type I second-degree AV block frequently results from increased parasympathetic tone or the effects of certain drugs. Coronary artery disease (CAD), inferior-wall myocardial infarction (MI), and rheumatic fever may increase parasympathetic tone and result in the arrhythmia. It may also be caused by cardiac medications, such as beta-adrenergic blockers, digoxin, and calcium channel blockers.

Clinical significance

Type I second-degree AV block may occur normally in an otherwise healthy person. Almost always transient, this type of block usually resolves when the underlying condition is corrected. Although an asymptomatic patient with

Type I second-degree AV block

+ Each successive impulse from SA node is delayed slightly longer than previous impulse
+ Pattern continues until impulse fails to be conducted to ventricles

Causes

+ Increased parasympathetic tone
+ Certain drugs
+ CAD
+ Inferior-wall MI
+ Rheumatic fever

Recognizing type I second-degree AV block

This rhythm strip illustrates type I second-degree atrioventricular (AV) block.

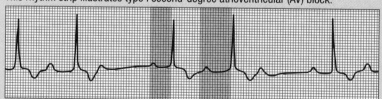

+ *Rhythm:* atrial — regular; ventricular — irregular
+ *Rate:* atrial — 80 beats/minute; ventricular — 50 beats/minute
+ *P wave:* normal
+ *PR interval:* progressively prolonged (see shaded areas)
+ *QRS complex:* 0.08 second
+ *T wave:* inverted
+ *QT interval:* 0.46 second
+ *Other:* Wenckebach pattern of grouped beats; the PR interval gets progressively longer until a QRS complex is dropped

this block has a good prognosis, the block may progress to a more serious form, especially if it occurs early in an MI.

ECG characteristics

ECG characteristics

+ *Rhythm*—atrial rhythm regular; ventricular rhythm irregular
+ *Rate*—atrial rate exceeds ventricular rate
+ *P wave*—normal size and configuration; followed by QRS complex, except for blocked P wave
+ *PR interval*—progressively longer with each cycle until P wave appears without QRS complex
+ *QRS complex*—duration usually remains within normal limits; periodically absent

Rhythm: Atrial rhythm is regular, and the ventricular rhythm is irregular. The R-R interval shortens progressively until a P wave appears without a QRS complex. The cycle is then repeated.

Rate: The atrial rate exceeds the ventricular rate because of the nonconducted beats, but both usually remain within normal limits.

P wave: Normal size and configuration; each P wave is followed by a QRS complex except for the blocked P wave.

PR interval: The PR interval is progressively longer with each cycle until a P wave appears without a QRS complex. The variation in delay from cycle to cycle is typically slight. The PR interval after the nonconducted beat is shorter than the interval preceding it. The phrase commonly used to describe this pattern is *long, longer, dropped.*

QRS complex: Duration usually remains within normal limits because the block commonly occurs at the level of the AV node. The complex is periodically absent.

T wave: Normal size and configuration.

QT interval: Usually within normal limits.

Other: The arrhythmia is usually distinguished by "group beating", referred to as the *footprints of Wenckebach.* K. Frederik Wenckebach was a Dutch internist who, at the turn of the century and long before the introduction of the ECG, described the two forms of what's now known as *second-degree AV block* by analyzing waves in the jugular venous pulse. Following the introduction of the ECG, German cardiologist Woldemar Mobitz clarified Wenckebach's findings, identifying two types of second-degree AV block, type I and type II.

Signs and symptoms

Signs and symptoms

+ Usually asymptomatic, but may show signs and symptoms of decreased cardiac output
+ Especially pronounced if ventricular rate is slow

Usually asymptomatic, a patient with type I second-degree AV block may show signs and symptoms of decreased cardiac output, such as light-headedness or hypotension. Symptoms may be especially pronounced if the ventricular rate is slow.

Interventions

Interventions

+ Rarely needed because patient is usually asymptomatic
+ For symptomatic patient, transcutaneous pacemaker until arrhythmia resolves
+ For patient with serious signs and symptoms related to low heart rate, atropine to improve AV conduction

Treatment is rarely needed because the patient is generally asymptomatic. A transcutaneous pacemaker may be required for a symptomatic patient until the arrhythmia resolves. (See *Bradycardia algorithm,* page 53, in chapter 4.) For a patient with serious signs and symptoms related to a low heart rate, atropine may be used to improve AV node conduction.

When caring for a patient with this block, assess the tolerance for the rhythm and the need for treatment to improve cardiac output. Evaluate the patient for possible causes of the block, including the use of certain medications or the presence of myocardial ischemia.

Check the ECG frequently to see if a more severe type of AV block develops. Make sure the patient has a patent I.V. line. Provide patient teaching about a temporary pacemaker if indicated.

TYPE II SECOND-DEGREE AV BLOCK

Type II second-degree AV block (also known as *Mobitz II block*) is less common than type I, but more serious. It occurs when impulses from the SA node occasionally fail to conduct to the ventricles. This form of second-degree AV block occurs below the level of the AV node, either at the bundle of His, or more commonly at the bundle branches.

One of the hallmarks of this type of block is that, unlike type I second-degree AV block, the PR interval doesn't lengthen before a dropped beat. (See *Recognizing type II second-degree AV block.*) In addition, more than one non-conducted beat can occur in succession.

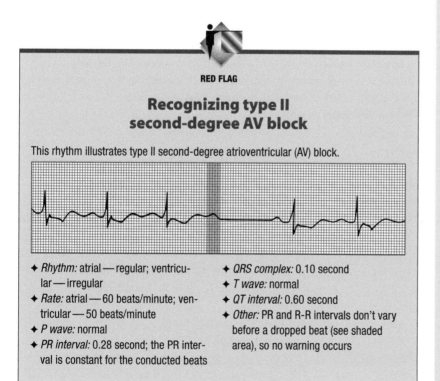

RED FLAG

Recognizing type II second-degree AV block

This rhythm illustrates type II second-degree atrioventricular (AV) block.

+ *Rhythm:* atrial — regular; ventricular — irregular
+ *Rate:* atrial — 60 beats/minute; ventricular — 50 beats/minute
+ *P wave:* normal
+ *PR interval:* 0.28 second; the PR interval is constant for the conducted beats
+ *QRS complex:* 0.10 second
+ *T wave:* normal
+ *QT interval:* 0.60 second
+ *Other:* PR and R-R intervals don't vary before a dropped beat (see shaded area), so no warning occurs

Interventions
(continued)

+ Monitor ECG to detect progression to more serious form of block

Type II second-degree AV block

+ Less common (than type I) but more serious
+ Impulses from SA node occasionally fail to conduct to ventricles
+ Occurs at bundle of His or at bundle branches (more common site)
+ PR interval doesn't lengthen before dropped beat (unlike type I)

Causes

+ Anterior-wall MI
+ Degenerative changes in conduction system
+ Severe CAD

Causes

Unlike type I second-degree AV block, type II second-degree AV block rarely results from increased parasympathetic tone or drug effect. Because the arrhythmia is usually associated with organic heart disease, it's usually associated with a poorer prognosis, and complete heart block may develop.

Type II second-degree AV block is commonly caused by an anterior-wall MI, degenerative changes in the conduction system, or severe CAD. The arrhythmia indicates a conduction disturbance at the level of the bundle of His or bundle branches.

Clinical significance

Unlike type I second-degree AV block, type II second-degree AV block rarely results from increased parasympathetic tone or drug effect. As a result, this type of block is usually associated with a poorer prognosis and a greater probability that complete heart block may develop.

In type II second-degree AV block, the ventricular rate tends to be slower than in type I. In addition, cardiac output tends to be lower and symptoms are more likely to appear, particularly if the sinus rhythm is slow and the ratio of conducted beats to dropped beats is low such as 2:1.

ECG characteristics

+ *Rhythm*—atrial rhythm regular; ventricular rhythm varied
+ *Rate*—atrial rate usually within normal limits; ventricular rate slower than atrial rate
+ *P wave*—normal in size and configuration; not always followed by QRS complex
+ *PR interval*—within normal limits or prolonged, but usually always constant for conducted beats
+ *QRS complex*—duration within normal limits, if block occurs at bundle of His; widened, if block occurs at bundle branches

ECG characteristics

Rhythm: The atrial rhythm is regular. The ventricular rhythm can be regular or irregular. Pauses correspond to the dropped beat. When the block is intermittent or when the conduction ratio is variable, the rhythm is often irregular. When a constant conduction ratio occurs, for example, 2:1 or 3:1, the rhythm is regular.

Rate: The atrial rate is usually within normal limits. The ventricular rate, slower than the atrial rate, may be within normal limits.

P wave: The P wave is normal in size and configuration, but some P waves aren't followed by a QRS complex. The R-R interval containing a nonconducted P wave equals two normal R-R intervals.

PR interval: The PR interval is within normal limits or prolonged but generally always constant for the conducted beats.

QRS complex: Duration is within normal limits if the block occurs at the bundle of His. If the block occurs at the bundle branches, however, the QRS will be widened and display the features of bundle-branch block. The complex is absent periodically.

T wave: Usually of normal size and configuration.

QT interval: Usually within normal limits.

Other: The PR and R-R intervals don't vary before a dropped beat, so no warning occurs. For a dropped beat to occur, there must be complete block

Distinguishing nonconducted PACs from type II second-degree AV block

An isolated P wave that doesn't conduct through to the ventricle (P wave without a QRS complex following it; see shaded areas) may occur with a nonconducted premature atrial contraction (PAC) or may indicate type II second-degree atrioventricular (AV) block. Mistakenly identifying AV block as nonconducted PACs may have serious consequences. The latter is generally benign; the former can be life-threatening.

NONCONDUCTED PAC
If the P-P interval, including the extra P wave, isn't constant, it's a nonconducted PAC.

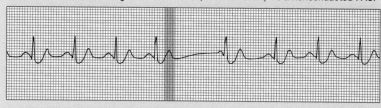

TYPE II SECOND-DEGREE AV BLOCK
If the P-P interval is constant, including the extra P wave, it's type II second-degree AV block.

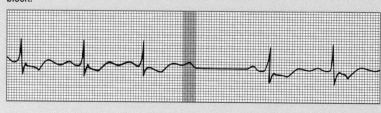

in one bundle branch with intermittent interruption in conduction in the other bundle as well. As a result, this type of second-degree AV block is commonly associated with a wide QRS complex. However, when the block occurs at the bundle of His, the QRS may be narrow since ventricular conduction is undisturbed in beats that aren't blocked.

It may be difficult to distinguish nonconducted premature atrial contractions (PACs) from type II second-degree AV block. (See *Distinguishing nonconducted PACs from type II second-degree AV block.*)

Signs and symptoms

Most patients who experience occasional dropped beats remain asymptomatic as long as cardiac output is maintained. As the number of dropped

Signs and symptoms
✦ Asymptomatic with occasional dropped beats (as long as cardiac output is maintained)

Signs and symptoms
(continued)
+ Symptomatic (as dropped beats increase), exhibiting signs and symptoms of decreased cardiac output

Interventions
+ Transvenous pacemaker insertion, if no signs and symptoms of low heart rate; or, continuous monitoring, with transcutaneous pacemaker readily available
+ Transcutaneous pacing or I.V. dopamine, epinephrine, or atropine to increase heart rate, if signs and symptoms of bradycardia
+ Atropine must be used cautiously as it can worsen ischemia during MI
+ May also require permanent pacemaker (can use temporary until permanent can be inserted)

beats increases, the patient may experience signs and symptoms of decreased cardiac output, including fatigue, dyspnea, chest pain, or light-headedness. On physical examination, you may note hypotension and a slow pulse, with a regular or irregular rhythm.

Interventions

If the patient doesn't experience serious signs and symptoms related to the low heart rate, he may be prepared for transvenous pacemaker insertion. Alternatively, the patient may be continuously monitored, with a transcutaneous pacemaker readily available.

If the patient is experiencing serious signs and symptoms due to bradycardia, treatment goals include improving cardiac output by increasing the heart rate. Transcutaneous pacing, I.V. dopamine, I.V. epinephrine or I.V. atropine may be used to increase cardiac output. (See *Bradycardia algorithm,* page 53, chapter 4.) Use atropine cautiously because it can worsen ischemia during an MI and may induce ventricular tachycardia or fibrillation in patients with this form of second-degree AV block and complete heart block.

Because this form of second-degree AV block occurs below the level of the AV node — either at the bundle of His or, more commonly, at the bundle branches — transcutaneous pacing should be initiated quickly, when indicated. For this reason, type II second-degree AV block also may require placement of a permanent pacemaker. A temporary pacemaker may be used until a permanent pacemaker can be inserted.

When caring for a patient with type II second-degree block, assess tolerance for the rhythm and the need for treatment to improve cardiac output. Evaluate for possible correctable causes such as ischemia.

Keep the patient on bed rest, if indicated, to reduce myocardial oxygen demands. Administer oxygen therapy as ordered. Observe the patient's cardiac rhythm for progression to a more severe form of AV block. Teach the patient and family about the use of pacemakers if the patient requires one.

Third-degree AV block
+ Complete absence of impulse conduction between atria and ventricles
+ Atrial rate generally faster than ventricular rate
+ Occurs at level of AV node, bundle of His, or bundle branches

THIRD-DEGREE ATRIOVENTRICULAR BLOCK

Also called *complete heart block,* third-degree atrioventricular (AV) block indicates the complete absence of impulse conduction between the atria and ventricles. In complete heart block, the atrial rate is generally faster than the ventricular rate.

Third-degree AV block may occur at the level of the AV node, the bundle of His, or the bundle branches. The patient's treatment and prognosis vary depending on the anatomic level of the block.

RED FLAG

Recognizing third-degree AV block

This rhythm strip illustrates third-degree atrioventricular (AV) block:

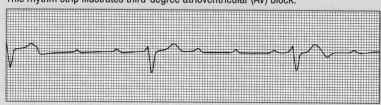

◆ *Rhythm:* regular
◆ *Rate:* atrial — 90 beats/minute; ventricular — 30 beats/minute
◆ *P wave:* normal
◆ *PR interval:* varied

◆ *QRS complex:* 0.16 second
◆ *T wave:* normal
◆ *QT interval:* 0.56 second
◆ *Other:* P waves occur without a QRS complex

When third-degree AV block occurs at the level of the AV node, ventricular depolarization is typically initiated by a junctional escape pacemaker. This pacemaker is usually stable with a rate of 40 to 60 beats/minute. (See *Recognizing third-degree AV block*.) The sequence of ventricular depolarization is usually normal because the block is located above the bifurcation of the bundle of His, which results in a normal-appearing QRS complex.

On the other hand, when third-degree AV block occurs at the infranodal level, a block involving the right and left bundle branches is most commonly the cause. In this case, extensive disease exists in the infranodal conduction system, and the only available escape mechanism is located distal to the site of block in the ventricle. This unstable, ventricular escape pacemaker has a slow intrinsic rate of less than 40 beats/minute. Because these depolarizations originate in the ventricle, the QRS complex will have a wide and bizarre appearance.

CAUSES

Third-degree AV block occurring at the anatomic level of the AV node can result from increased parasympathetic tone associated with inferior wall myocardial infarction (MI), AV node damage, or toxic effects of such drugs as digoxin and propranolol.

Third-degree AV block
(continued)

◆ If block occurs at level of AV node, ventricular depolarization typically initiated by junctional escape pacemaker
◆ If block occurs at infranodal level, a block involving right and left bundle branches is likely cause
◆ Unstable, ventricular escape pacemaker has slow intrinsic rate of < 40 beats/minute

Causes

◆ Increased parasympathetic tone associated with inferior wall MI, AV node damage, or toxic effects of certain drugs, if block occurs at anatomic level of AV node
◆ Extensive anterior MI, if block occurs at infranodal level

Third-degree AV block occurring at the infranodal level is frequently associated with extensive anterior MI. It generally isn't the result of increases in parasympathetic tone or drug effect.

CLINICAL SIGNIFICANCE

Third-degree AV block occurring at the AV node, with a junctional escape rhythm, is usually transient and generally associated with a favorable prognosis. In third-degree AV block at the infranodal level, however, the pacemaker is unstable and episodes of ventricular asystole are common. Third-degree AV block at this level is generally associated with a less favorable prognosis.

Because the ventricular rate in third-degree AV block can be slow and the decrease in cardiac output so significant, the arrhythmia usually results in a life-threatening situation. In addition, the loss of AV synchrony results in the loss of atrial kick, which further decreases cardiac output.

ECG characteristics

+ *Rhythm*—atrial and ventricular rhythms usually regular
+ *Rate*—atrial rate (under control of SA node) at 60 to 100 beats/minute; with intranodal block, ventricular rate usually at 40 to 60 beats/minute; with intranodal block, ventricular rate usually < 40 beats/minute
+ *P wave*—normal size and configuration
+ *PR interval*—unmeasurable (and not applicable)
+ *QRS complex*—depends on location of escape mechanism (if block occurs at level of AV node or bundle of His, appears normal; if block occurs at level of bundle branches, widened)

ECG CHARACTERISTICS

Rhythm: Atrial and ventricular rhythms are usually regular.
Rate: Acting independently, the atria, generally under the control of the sinoatrial (SA) node, tend to maintain a regular rate of 60 to 100 beats/minute. The atrial rate exceeds the ventricular rate. With intranodal block, the ventricular rate is usually 40 to 60 beats/minute (a junctional escape rhythm). With infranodal block, the ventricular rate is usually below 40 beats/minute (a ventricular escape rhythm).
P wave: The P wave is normal in size and configuration. Some P waves may be buried in QRS complexes or T waves.
PR interval: Not applicable or measurable because the atria and ventricles are depolarized from different pacemakers and beat independently of each other.
QRS complex: Configuration depends on the location of the escape mechanism and origin of ventricular depolarization. When the block occurs at the level of the AV node or bundle of His, the QRS complex will appear normal. When the block occurs at the level of the bundle branches, the QRS will be widened.
T wave: Normal size and configuration unless the QRS complex originates in the ventricle.
QT interval: May be within normal limits.
Other: None.

SIGNS AND SYMPTOMS

Most patients with third-degree AV block experience significant signs and symptoms, including severe fatigue, dyspnea, chest pain, light-headedness, changes in mental status, and changes in the level of consciousness. Hypotension, pallor, and diaphoresis may also occur. The peripheral pulse rate will be slow, but the rhythm will be regular.

A few patients will be relatively free of symptoms, complaining only that they can't tolerate exercise and that they're typically tired for no apparent reason. The severity of symptoms depends to a large extent on the resulting ventricular rate and the patient's ability to compensate for decreased cardiac output.

INTERVENTIONS

If the patient is experiencing serious signs and symptoms related to the low heart rate, or if the patient's condition seems to be deteriorating, interventions may include transcutaneous pacing or I.V. atropine, dopamine, or epinephrine. Atropine isn't indicated for third-degree AV block with new wide QRS complexes. In such cases, a permanent pacemaker is indicated because atropine rarely increases sinus rate and AV node conduction when AV block is at the His-Purkinje level.

Asymptomatic patients in third-degree AV block should be prepared for insertion of a transvenous temporary pacemaker until a decision is made about the need for a permanent pacemaker. If symptoms develop, a transcutaneous pacemaker should be used until the transvenous pacemaker is placed.

Because third-degree AV block occurring at the infranodal level is usually associated with extensive anterior MI, patients are more likely to have permanent third-degree AV block, which most likely requires insertion of a permanent pacemaker.

Third-degree AV block occurring at the anatomic level of the AV node can result from increased parasympathetic tone associated with an inferior wall MI. As a result, the block is more likely to be short-lived. In these patients, the decision to insert a permanent pacemaker is often delayed to assess how well the conduction system recovers.

When caring for a patient with third-degree heart block, immediately assess the patient's tolerance of the rhythm and the need for interventions to support cardiac output and relieve symptoms. Make sure that the patient has

Signs and symptoms

+ Severe fatigue, dyspnea, chest pain, light-headedness, altered mental status and LOC, hypotension, pallor, and diaphoresis
+ Peripheral pulse rate slow, but rhythm regular
+ Occasionally asymptomatic, with complaints of not tolerating exercise and feeling tired

Interventions

+ Transcutaneous pacing or I.V. atropine, dopamine, or epinephrine, if signs and symptoms related to low heart rate or if patient's condition deteriorating
+ Permanent pacemaker (not atropine), if new wide QRS complexes
+ Prepare for transvenous temporary pacemaker (until decision is made regarding a permanent pacemaker), if asymptomatic

a patent I.V. line. Administer oxygen therapy as ordered. Evaluate for possible correctable causes of the arrhythmia, such as drugs or myocardial ischemia. Minimize the patient's activity and maintain bed rest.

 AGE CHANGE After repair of a ventricular septal defect, a child may require a permanent pacemaker if complete heart block develops. This arrhythmia may develop from interference with the bundle of His during surgery.

Electrolyte imbalances and drugs

This chapter reviews ECG characteristics associated with electrolyte imbalances and drugs.

Rhythm strips of patients with electrolyte imbalances, such as hyperkalemia, hypokalemia, hypercalcemia, and hypocalcemia, frequently show distinctive patterns. Patients taking such drugs as digoxin may also exhibit characteristic appearances on an ECG that can provide early warnings of drug toxicity. By recognizing some of these variations early, you may be able to identify and treat potentially dangerous conditions before they become serious.

Keep in mind, however, that the patient's ECG is only part of the clinical picture. Additional information, such as the patient's medical history, findings on physical examination, and additional diagnostic studies, will be necessary to confirm an initial diagnosis based on ECG analysis.

ELECTROLYTE IMBALANCES

Potassium and calcium ions play a major role in the electrical activity of the heart. Depolarization results from the exchange of these ions across the cell membrane. Changes in ion concentration can affect the heart's electrical activity and, as a result, the patient's ECG. This section examines ECG effects from high and low potassium and calcium levels.

Electrolyte imbalances
◆ Changes in potassium and calcium ions play major role in heart's electrical activity

Hyperkalemia
+ Elevation of serum potassium > 5 mEq/L

HYPERKALEMIA

Potassium, the most plentiful intracellular cation (positively charged electrolyte), contributes to many important cellular functions. Most of the body's potassium content is located in the cells. The intracellular fluid (ICF) concentration of potassium is 150 to 160 mEq/L; the extracellular fluid (ECF) concentration, 3.5 to 4.5 mEq/L. Many symptoms associated with potassium imbalance result from changes in this ratio of ICF to ECF potassium concentration. Hyperkalemia is generally defined as an elevation of serum potassium above 5 mEq/L.

Causes
+ Increased intake of potassium through diet and I.V. administration
+ Potassium shifting from ICF to ECF and occurring with changes in cell membrane permeability

CAUSES

+ An increased intake of potassium, including excessive dietary intake and I.V. administration of penicillin G, potassium supplements, or banked whole blood.
+ A shift of potassium from ICF to ECF occurring with changes in cell membrane permeability or damage, including extensive surgery, burns, massive crush injuries, cell hypoxia, acidosis, and insulin deficiency.
+ Decreased renal excretion, including renal failure, decreased production and secretion of aldosterone, Addison's disease, and use of potassium-sparing diuretics.

CLINICAL SIGNIFICANCE

When extracellular potassium concentrations increase without a significant change in intracellular potassium concentrations, the cell becomes less negative, or partially depolarized, and the resting cell membrane potential decreases. Mild elevations in extracellular potassium result in cells that repolarize faster and are more irritable.

More critical elevations in extracellular potassium result in an inability of cells to repolarize and respond to electrical stimuli. Cardiac standstill, or *asystole*, is the most serious consequence of severe hyperkalemia.

ECG characteristics
+ *Rhythm*—atrial and ventricular rhythms regular
+ *Rate*—atrial and ventricular rates within normal limits
+ *P wave*—low amplitude; wide and flattened; indiscernible
+ *PR interval*—normal or prolonged; unmeasurable if P wave undetectable

ECG CHARACTERISTICS

Rhythm: Atrial and ventricular rhythms are regular.
Rate: Atrial and ventricular rates are within normal limits.
P wave: In mild hyperkalemia, the amplitude is low; in moderate hyperkalemia, P waves are wide and flattened; in severe hyperkalemia, the P wave may be indiscernible.
PR interval: Normal or prolonged; not measurable if P wave can't be detected.

QRS complex: Widened because ventricular depolarization takes longer.
ST segment: May be elevated in severe hyperkalemia.
T wave: Tall, peaked; the classic and most striking feature of hyperkalemia.
QT interval: Shortened.
Other: Intraventricular conduction disturbances commonly occur. (See *ECG effects of hyperkalemia.*)

SIGNS AND SYMPTOMS

Mild hyperkalemia may cause neuromuscular irritability, including restlessness, intestinal cramping, diarrhea, and tingling lips and fingers. Severe hyperkalemia may cause loss of muscle tone, muscle weakness, and paralysis.

INTERVENTIONS

Treatment depends upon the severity of hyperkalemia and the patient's signs and symptoms. The underlying cause must be identified and the extracellular potassium concentration brought back to normal. Drug therapy to normalize potassium levels includes calcium gluconate to decrease neuromuscular irritability, insulin and glucose to facilitate the entry of potassium into the cell, and sodium bicarbonate to correct metabolic acidosis.

Oral or rectal administration of cation exchange resins, such as sodium polystyrene sulfonate, may be used to exchange sodium for potassium in the intestine. In the setting of renal failure or severe hyperkalemia, dialysis may be necessary to remove excess potassium. The patient's serum potassium levels should be monitored closely until they return to normal, and arrhythmias should be identified and managed appropriately.

ECG effects of hyperkalemia

The classic and most striking ECG feature of hyperkalemia is tall, peaked T waves. This rhythm strip shows a typical peaked T wave (shaded area).

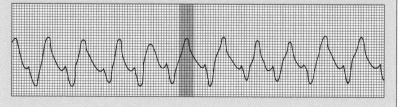

Hypokalemia
+ ECF concentration of potassium drops < 3.5 mEq/L

HYPOKALEMIA

Hypokalemia, or potassium deficiency, occurs when the extracellular fluid (ECF) concentration of potassium drops below 3.5 mEq/L, usually indicating a loss of total body potassium. The concentration of ECF potassium is so small that even minor changes in ECF potassium affect resting membrane potential.

Causes
+ Increased loss of body potassium
+ Increased entry of potassium into cells
+ Reduced potassium intake
+ GI and renal disorders
+ Diuretics (low serum magnesium concentration)
+ Excessive aldosterone secretion

CAUSES

Factors contributing to the development of hypokalemia include increased loss of body potassium, increased entry of potassium into cells, and reduced potassium intake. Shifts in potassium from the extracellular space to the intracellular space may be caused by alkalosis, especially respiratory alkalosis. Intracellular uptake of potassium is also increased by catecholamines. Although rare, dietary deficiency in the elderly may contribute to hypokalemia. The condition is also seen in patients with alcoholism or anorexia nervosa.

GI and renal disorders are the most common causes of potassium loss from body stores. GI losses of potassium are associated with laxative abuse, intestinal fistulae or drainage tubes, diarrhea, vomiting, and continuous nasogastric drainage.

Renal loss of potassium is related to increased secretion of potassium by the distal tubule. Diuretics, a low serum magnesium concentration, and excessive aldosterone secretion may cause urinary loss of potassium. In addition, several antibiotics, including gentamicin and amphotericin B, are known to cause hypokalemia.

CLINICAL SIGNIFICANCE

When extracellular potassium levels decrease rapidly and intracellular potassium concentration doesn't change, the resting membrane potential becomes more negative and the cell membrane becomes hyperpolarized. The cardiac effects of hypokalemia are related to these changes in membrane excitability. Ventricular repolarization is delayed because potassium contributes to the repolarization phase of the action potential. Hypokalemia can cause dangerous ventricular arrhythmias and increases the risk of digoxin toxicity.

ECG characteristics
+ *Rhythm*—atrial and ventricular rhythms regular
+ *Rate*—atrial and ventricular rates within normal limits
+ *P wave*—usually normal size and configuration; may become peaked in severe hypokalemia
+ *PR interval*—possibly prolonged

ECG CHARACTERISTICS

Rhythm: Atrial and ventricular rhythms are regular.
Rate: Atrial and ventricular rates are within normal limits.
P wave: Usually normal size and configuration but may become peaked in severe hypokalemia.
PR interval: May be prolonged.

QRS complex: Within normal limits or possibly widened; prolonged in severe hypokalemia.

QT interval: Usually indiscernible as the T wave flattens.

ST segment: Depressed.

T wave: Amplitude is decreased. The T wave becomes flat as the potassium level drops. In severe hypokalemia, it flattens completely and may become inverted. The T wave may also fuse with an increasingly prominent U wave.

Other: Amplitude of the U wave is increased, becoming more prominent as hypokalemia worsens and fusing with the T wave. (See *ECG effects of hypokalemia.*)

SIGNS AND SYMPTOMS

The most common symptoms of hypokalemia are caused by neuromuscular and cardiac effects, including smooth muscle atony, skeletal muscle weakness, and cardiac arrhythmias. Loss of smooth muscle tone results in constipation, intestinal distention, nausea, vomiting, anorexia, and paralytic ileus. Skeletal muscle weakness occurs first in the larger muscles of the arms and legs and eventually affects the diaphragm, causing respiratory arrest.

Cardiac effects of hypokalemia include arrhythmias, such as bradycardia, atrioventricular (AV) block, and paroxysmal atrial tachycardia. Delayed depolarization results in characteristic changes on the ECG.

INTERVENTIONS

The underlying causes of hypokalemia should be identified and corrected. Acid-base imbalances should be corrected, potassium losses replaced, and further losses prevented. Encourage intake of foods and fluids rich in potassium. Oral or I.V. potassium supplements may be administered. The patient's serum potassium levels should be monitored closely until they return to

ECG characteristics (continued)

✦ *QRS complex*—within normal limits or possibly widened; prolonged in severe hypokalemia
✦ *QT interval*—usually indiscernible as T wave flattens
✦ *ST segment*—depressed
✦ *T wave*—amplitude decreased; becomes flat in severe hypokalemia; may also fuse with U wave

Signs and symptoms

✦ Loss of smooth muscle tone, resulting in constipation, intestinal distention, nausea, vomiting, anorexia, and paralytic ileus
✦ Skeletal muscle weakness, affecting the diaphragm, leading to respiratory arrest
✦ Arrhythmias, including bradycardia, AV block, paroxysmal atrial tachycardia
✦ Delayed depolarization, resulting in changes on ECG

Interventions

✦ Identify and correct underlying causes
✦ Correct acid-base imbalances and replace potassium losses
✦ Monitor serum potassium levels and for development of arrhythmias

ECG effects of hypokalemia

As the serum potassium concentration drops, the T wave becomes flat and a U wave appears (shaded area). This rhythm strip shows typical ECG effects of hypokalemia.

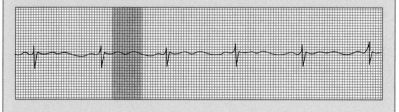

normal, and cardiac arrhythmias should be identified and managed appropriately.

Hypercalcemia
✦ Serum calcium concentration > 10.5 mg/dl

HYPERCALCEMIA

Most of the body's calcium stores (99%) are located in bone. The remainder is found in the plasma and body cells. Approximately 50% of plasma calcium is bound to plasma proteins. About 40% is found in the ionized or free form.

Calcium plays an important role in myocardial contractility. Ionized calcium is more important than plasma-bound calcium in physiologic functions. Hypercalcemia is usually defined as a serum calcium concentration greater than 10.5 mg/dl.

Causes
✦ Excessive vitamin D intake
✦ Bone metastasis and calcium resorption associated with cancers of breast, prostate, and cervix
✦ Hyperparathyroidism
✦ Sarcoidosis
✦ Parathyroid hormone–producing tumors

CAUSES

The most common causes of hypercalcemia include excess vitamin D intake; bone metastasis and calcium resorption associated with cancers of the breast, prostate, and cervix; hyperparathyroidism; sarcoidosis; and many parathyroid hormone–producing tumors.

CLINICAL SIGNIFICANCE

In hypercalcemia, calcium is found inside cells in greater abundance than normal. The cell membrane becomes refractory to depolarization as a result of a more positive action potential. This loss of cell membrane excitability causes many of the cardiac symptoms seen in patients with hypercalcemia.

Both ventricular depolarization and repolarization are accelerated. The patient may experience bradyarrhythmias and varying degrees of atrioventricular block.

ECG characteristics
✦ *Rhythm*—atrial and ventricular rhythms regular
✦ *Rate*—atrial and ventricular rates within normal limits
✦ *P wave*—normal size and configuration
✦ *PR interval*—possibly prolonged
✦ *QRS complex*—Within normal limits; possibly prolonged
✦ *QT interval*—shortened
✦ *ST segment*—shortened
✦ *T wave*—normal size and configuration; possibly depressed

ECG CHARACTERISTICS

Rhythm: Atrial and ventricular rhythms are regular.
Rate: Atrial and ventricular rates are within normal limits, but bradycardia can occur.
P wave: Normal size and configuration.
PR interval: May be prolonged.
QRS complex: Within normal limits, but may be prolonged.
QT interval: Shortened.
ST segment: Shortened.
T wave: Normal size and configuration; may be depressed.
Other: None. (See *ECG effects of hypercalcemia.*)

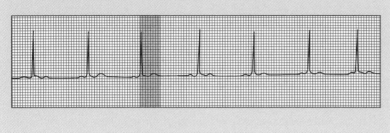

ECG effects of hypercalcemia

Increased serum concentrations of calcium cause shortening of the QT interval as shown (shaded area) in this ECG rhythm strip.

Signs and symptoms

Common signs and symptoms of hypercalcemia include anorexia, nausea, constipation, lethargy, fatigue, and weakness. Behavioral changes may also occur. Renal calculi may form as precipitates of calcium salts, and impaired renal function frequently occurs. A reciprocal decrease in serum phosphate levels often accompanies elevated levels of serum calcium.

Interventions

Treatment of hypercalcemia focuses on identifying and managing the underlying cause and is guided by the severity of the patient's symptoms. The administration of oral phosphate is usually effective as long as renal function is normal. In more critical situations, I.V. administration of large volumes of normal saline solution may enhance renal excretion of calcium. Patients in renal failure may need dialysis. Corticosteroids and calcitonin may be used to treat hypercalcemia.

HYPOCALCEMIA

Hypocalcemia occurs when the serum calcium level is below 8.5 mg/dl

Causes

Hypocalcemia may be related to decreases in parathyroid hormone and vitamin D, inadequate intestinal absorption, blood administration, or deposition of ionized calcium into soft tissue or bone.

Inadequate dietary intake of green, leafy vegetables or dairy products may result in a nutritional deficiency of calcium. Excessive dietary intake of phosphorus binds with calcium and prevents calcium absorption. The citrate so-

Signs and symptoms
◆ Anorexia, nausea, constipation, lethargy, fatigue, and weakness
◆ Renal calculi, resulting in impaired renal function

Interventions
◆ Identify and manage underlying cause
◆ Oral phosphate usually effective if renal function is normal
◆ I.V. normal saline solution (large volumes) may enhance renal excretion of calcium if more critical
◆ Dialysis for renal failure
◆ Corticosteroids and calcitonin

Hypocalcemia
◆ Serum calcium level < 8.5 mg/dl

Causes
◆ Decreases in parathyroid hormone and vitamin D
◆ Inadequate intestinal absorption, blood administration, or deposition of ionized calcium into soft tissue or bone
◆ Inadequate intake of green, leafy vegetables or dairy

lution used in storing whole blood binds with calcium, frequently resulting in hypocalcemia. Pancreatitis decreases ionized calcium, and neoplastic bone metastases decrease serum calcium levels.

Decreased intestinal absorption of calcium is caused by vitamin D deficiency, either from inadequate vitamin D intake or insufficient exposure to sunlight. Other causes of hypocalcemia include malabsorption of fats, removal of the parathyroid glands, metabolic or respiratory alkalosis, and hypoalbuminemia.

CLINICAL SIGNIFICANCE

Hypocalcemia causes an increase in neuromuscular excitability. Partial depolarization of nerves and muscle cells result from a decrease in threshold potential. As a result, a smaller stimulus is needed to initiate an action potential. Characteristic ECG changes are a result of prolonged ventricular depolarization and decreased cardiac contractility.

ECG CHARACTERISTICS

Rhythm: Atrial and ventricular rhythms are regular.
Rate: Atrial and ventricular rates are within normal limits.
P wave: Normal size and configuration.
PR interval: Within normal limits.
QRS complex: Within normal limits.
QT interval: Prolonged.
ST segment: Prolonged.
T wave: Normal size and configuration, but may become flat or inverted.
Other: None. (See *ECG effects of hypocalcemia.*)

ECG characteristics

+ *Rhythm*—atrial and ventricular rhythms regular
+ *Rate*—atrial and ventricular rates within normal limits
+ *P wave*—normal size and configuration
+ *QRS complex*—within normal limits
+ *QT interval*—prolonged
+ *ST segment*—prolonged
+ *T wave*—normal size and configuration; possibly flat or inverted

ECG effects of hypocalcemia

Decreased serum concentrations of calcium prolong the QT interval, as shown (shaded area) in this ECG rhythm strip.

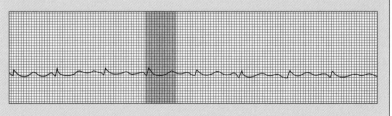

SIGNS AND SYMPTOMS

Symptoms of hypocalcemia include hyperreflexia, carpopedal spasm, confusion, and circumoral and digital paresthesia. Hyperactive bowel sounds and intestinal cramping may also occur. Severe symptoms include tetany, seizures, respiratory arrest, and death. Clinical signs indicating hypocalcemia include Trousseau's sign and Chvostek's sign.

INTERVENTIONS

Treatment should focus on identifying and managing the underlying causes of hypocalcemia. Severe symptoms require emergency treatment with I.V. calcium gluconate. Serum calcium levels should be monitored and oral calcium replacement initiated when possible. Cardiac arrhythmias need to be identified and managed appropriately. Long-term management of hypocalcemia includes decreasing phosphate intake.

CARDIAC DRUGS

Almost half a million U.S. residents die each year from cardiac arrhythmias; countless others experience symptoms and lifestyle modifications. Along with other treatments, cardiac drugs can help alleviate symptoms, control heart rate and rhythm, decrease preload and afterload, and prolong life.

Antiarrhythmics affect the movement of ions across the cell membrane and alter the electrophysiology of the cardiac cell. These drugs are classified according to their effect on the cell's electrical activity (action potential) and their mechanism of action. Because the drugs can cause changes in the myocardial action potential, characteristic ECG changes can occur.

The classification system divides antiarrhythmic drugs into four major classes based on their dominant mechanism of action: class I, class II, class III, and class IV. Class I antiarrhythmics are further divided into class IA, class IB, and class IC.

Certain antiarrhythmics can't be classified specifically into one group. For example, sotalol possesses characteristics of both class II and class III drugs. Still other drugs, such as adenosine, digoxin, atropine, epinephrine, and magnesium, don't fit into the classification system at all. Despite its limitations, the classification system is helpful in understanding how antiarrhythmics prevent and treat arrhythmias.

This section reviews ECG changes that result when patients take therapeutic doses of antiarrhythmics (separated by classification) and digoxin. When drug levels are toxic, ECG changes are typically exaggerated.

Signs and symptoms

✦ Hyperreflexia, carpopedal spasm, confusion, circumoral and digital paresthesia, hyperactive bowel sounds, intestinal cramping
✦ Tetany, seizures, respiratory arrest (severe)

Interventions

✦ Treat underlying causes
✦ I.V. calcium gluconate for severe symptoms
✦ Monitor serum calcium levels and for development of arrhythmias

---

Cardiac drugs

Antiarrhythmics
✦ Classified according to their effect on cell's electrical activity and their mechanism of action
✦ Can cause changes in myocardial action potential resulting in characteristic ECG changes
✦ Divided into four major classes: class I, class II, class III, and class IV
✦ Class I further divided into class IA, class IB, and class IC
✦ Certain drugs can't be classified specifically into one group
✦ Drugs such as adenosine, digoxin, atropine, epinephrine, and magnesium can't even be classified

Class I antiarrhythmics

+ Block influx of sodium into cell during phase 0 of action potential
+ Also called *sodium channel blockers* or *fast channel blockers*
+ Often subdivided into A, B, and C

Class IA

+ Includes disopyramide, procainamide, and quinidine; lengthen action potential duration

ECG characteristics
+ *QRS complex*—slightly widened; increased widening early sign of toxicity
+ *T wave*—possibly flattened or inverted
+ *U wave*—possibly present
+ *QT interval*—prolonged, possibly resulting in polymorphic ventricular tachycardia

Class IB

+ Includes phenytoin, lidocaine, mexiletine, and tocainide; interact with sodium channels, slowing phase 0 of action potential and shortening phase 3

ECG characteristics
+ *PR interval*—slightly shortened (possibly)
+ *QT interval*—shortened

CLASS I ANTIARRHYTHMICS

Class I drugs block the influx of sodium into the cell during phase 0 of the action potential. Because phase 0 is also referred to as the sodium channel or fast channel, these drugs may also be called *sodium channel blockers* or *fast channel blockers*. Class I drugs are frequently subdivided into three groups—A, B, and C—according to their interactions with cardiac sodium channels or the drug's effects on the duration of the action potential.

CLASS IA

Class IA drugs include disopyramide, procainamide, and quinidine. These drugs lengthen the duration of the action potential, and their interaction with the sodium channels is classified as intermediate. As a result, conductivity is reduced and repolarization is prolonged.

ECG characteristics

Rhythm strip characteristics for a patient taking an antiarrhythmic vary according to the drug's classification. Variations for class IA drugs include:
+ *QRS complex:* Slightly widened; increased widening is an early sign of toxicity.
+ *T wave:* May be flattened or inverted.
+ *U wave:* May be present.
+ *QT interval:* Prolonged.
+ Because these drugs prolong the QT interval, the patient is prone to polymorphic ventricular tachycardia. (See *ECG effects of class IA antiarrhythmics.*)

CLASS IB

Class IB agents include phenytoin, lidocaine, mexiletine, and tocainide. These agents interact rapidly with sodium channels, slowing phase 0 of the action potential and shortening phase 3. The drugs in this class are effective in suppressing ventricular ectopy.

ECG characteristics

When a patient is taking a class IB antiarrhythmic, check for these ECG changes:
+ *PR interval:* May be slightly shortened.
+ *QT interval:* Shortened. (See *ECG effects of class IB antiarrhythmics.*)

ECG effects of class IA antiarrhythmics

Class IA antiarrhythmics—such as quinidine and procainamide—affect the cardiac cycle in specific ways and lead to specific ECG changes, as shown here. Class IA antiarrhythmics:

✦ block sodium influx during phase 0, which depresses the rate of depolarization
✦ prolong repolarization and the duration of the action potential
✦ lengthen the refractory period
✦ decrease contractility.

ECG characteristics of class IA antiarrhythmics:

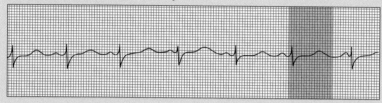

✦ *QRS complex:* slightly widened   ✦ *QT interval:* prolonged (shaded area)

ECG effects of class IB antiarrhythmics

Class IB antiarrhythmics—such as lidocaine and tocainide—may affect the QRS complex, as shown on the rhythm strip here. The drugs may also:
✦ block sodium influx during phase 0, which depresses the rate of depolarization
✦ shorten repolarization and the duration of the action potential
✦ suppress ventricular automaticity in ischemic tissue.

ECG characteristics of class IB antiarrhythmics:

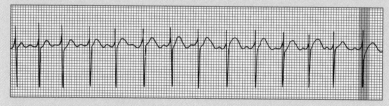

✦ *PR interval:* may be slightly shortened   ✦ *QRS complex:* slightly widened (shaded area)

ECG effects of class IC antiarrhythmics

Class IC antiarrhythmics—such as flecainide, propafenone and moricizine—exert particular actions on the cardiac cycle and lead to specific ECG changes, as shown here. Class IC antiarrhythmics block sodium influx during phase 0, which depresses the rate of depolarization. The drugs exert no effect on repolarization or the duration of the action potential.

ECG characteristics of class IC antiarrhythmics:

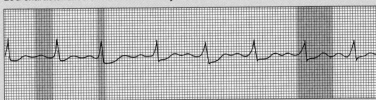

+ *PR interval:* prolonged (shaded area above left)
+ *QRS complex:* widened (shaded area above center)
+ *QT interval:* prolonged (shaded area above right)

Class IC

+ Include flecainide, propafenone, and moricizine; interact with sodium channels, markedly slowing phase 0 and decreasing conduction

ECG characteristics
+ *PR interval*—prolonged
+ *QRS complex*—widened
+ *QT interval*—prolonged

Class II antiarrhythmics

+ Reduce adrenergic activity in heart

CLASS IC

Class IC agents, including flecainide and propafenone, and moricizine (shares properties of classes IA, IB, and IC) may minimally increase or have no effect on the action potential duration. Class IC drugs interact slowly with sodium channels. Phase 0 is markedly slowed and conduction is decreased.

These agents are generally reserved for refractory arrhythmias because they may cause or worsen arrhythmias.

ECG characteristics

When a patient is taking a class IC antiarrhythmic, look for these ECG changes:
+ *PR interval:* Prolonged.
+ *QRS complex:* Widened.
+ *QT interval:* Prolonged. (See *ECG effects of class IC antiarrhythmics.*)

CLASS II ANTIARRHYTHMICS

Class II antiarrhythmics include drugs that reduce adrenergic activity in the heart. Beta-adrenergic antagonists, also called *beta blockers,* are class II antiarrhythmics and include such drugs as acebutolol, esmolol and propranolol. Beta-adrenergic antagonists block beta receptors in the sympathetic nervous system. As a result, phase 4 depolarization is diminished, which leads to depressed automaticity of the sinoatrial node and increased atrial and atrioventricular node refractory periods.

Class II drugs are used to treat supraventricular and ventricular arrhythmias, especially those caused by excess circulating catecholamines. Beta-adrenergic blockers are classified according to their effects. Beta$_1$-adrenergic blockers decrease heart rate, contractility, and conductivity. Beta$_2$-adrenergic blockers may cause vasoconstriction and bronchospasm because beta$_2$ receptors relax smooth muscle in the bronchi and blood vessels.

Beta-adrenergic blockers that block only beta$_1$ receptors are referred to as *cardioselective.* Those that block both beta$_1$- and beta$_2$-receptor activity are referred to as *noncardioselective.*

ECG CHARACTERISTICS

When a patient is taking a class II antiarrhythmic, you may see these ECG changes:
+ *Rate:* Atrial and ventricular rates are decreased.
+ *PR interval:* Slightly prolonged.
+ *QT interval:* Slightly shortened. (See *ECG effects of class II antiarrhythmics.*)

Class II antiarrhythmics (continued)

+ Include acebutolol, esmolol, and propranolol, which block beta receptors in sympathetic nervous system, resulting in diminished phase 4 depolarization
+ Those that block only beta$_1$ receptors (cardioselective); those that block beta$_1$- and beta$_2$- receptors (noncardioselective)

ECG characteristics

+ *Rate*—atrial and ventricular rates decreased
+ *PR interval*—slightly prolonged
+ *QT interval*—slightly shortened

ECG effects of class II antiarrhythmics

Class II antiarrhythmics—including such beta-adrenergic blockers as propranolol, esmolol, and acebutolol—exert particular actions on the cardiac cycle and lead to specific ECG changes, as shown here. Class II antiarrhythmics:
+ depress sinoatrial node automaticity
+ shorten the duration of the action potential
+ increase the refractory period of atrial and atrioventricular junctional tissues, which slows conduction
+ inhibit sympathetic activity.

ECG characteristics of class II antiarrhythmics:

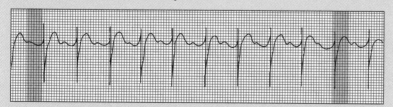

+ *PR interval:* slightly prolonged (shaded area above left)
+ *QT interval:* slightly shortened (shaded area above right)

Class III antiarrhythmics

◆ Prolong action potential duration, resulting in prolonged effective refractory period
◆ Block movement of potassium during phase 3 of action potential
◆ Include amiodarone, dofetilide, ibutilide, and sotalol

ECG characteristics

◆ *PR interval*—prolonged
◆ *QRS complex*—widened
◆ *QT interval*—prolonged

CLASS III ANTIARRHYTHMICS

Class III drugs prolong the action potential duration, which, in turn, prolongs the effective refractory period. Class III drugs are called *potassium channel blockers* because they block the movement of potassium during phase 3 of the action potential. Drugs in this class include amiodarone, dofetilide, ibutilide, and sotalol (a nonselective beta-adrenergic blocker with mainly class III properties). All class III drugs have proarrhythmic potential.

ECG CHARACTERISTICS

When a patient is taking a class III antiarrhythmic, you may see these ECG changes:
◆ *PR interval:* Prolonged.
◆ *QRS complex:* Widened.
◆ *QT interval:* Prolonged. (See *ECG effects of class III antiarrhythmics.*)

ECG effects of class III antiarrhythmics

Class III antiarrhythmics—such as amiodarone, sotalol, and ibutilide—affect the cardiac cycle and cause the changes shown here on an ECG rhythm strip. Class III antiarrhythmics:
◆ block potassium movement during phase 3
◆ increase the duration of the action potential
◆ prolong the effective refractory period.

ECG characteristics of class III antiarrhythmics:

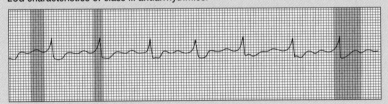

◆ *PR interval:* prolonged (shaded area above left)
◆ *QRS complex:* widened (shaded area above center)
◆ *QT interval:* prolonged (shaded area above right)

CLASS IV ANTIARRHYTHMICS

Class IV drugs block the movement of calcium during phase 2 of the action potential. Because phase 2 is also called the *calcium channel* or the *slow channel,* drugs that affect phase 2 are also known as *calcium channel blockers* or *slow channel blockers.* These drugs slow conduction and increase the refractory period of calcium-dependent tissues, including the atrioventricular node. Drugs in this class include verapamil and diltiazem.

 AGE CHANGE Administer diltiazem cautiously in the older adult because the half-life of the drug may be prolonged. Be especially careful if the older adult also has heart failure or impaired hepatic or renal function.

ECG CHARACTERISTICS

When a patient is taking a class IV antiarrhythmic, check for these ECG changes:

✦ *Rate:* Atrial and ventricular rates are decreased.
✦ *PR interval:* Prolonged. (See *ECG effects of class IV antiarrhythmics.*)

Class IV antiarrhythmics

✦ Block movement of calcium during phase 2 of action potential
✦ Slow conduction and increase refractory period of calcium-dependent tissues
✦ Include verapamil and diltiazem

ECG characteristics

✦ *Rate*—atrial and ventricular rates decreased
✦ *PR interval*—prolonged

ECG effects of class IV antiarrhythmics

Class IV antiarrhythmics—including such calcium channel blockers as verapamil and diltiazem—affect the cardiac cycle in specific ways and may lead to a prolonged PR interval as shown here on an ECG rhythm strip. Class IV antiarrhythmics:
✦ block calcium movement during phase 2
✦ prolong the conduction time and increase the refractory period in the atrioventricular node
✦ decrease contractility.

ECG characteristics of class IV antiarrhythmics:

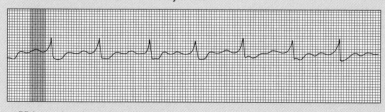

✦ *PR interval:* prolonged (shaded area)

Digoxin

✦ Works by inhibiting the enzyme, adenosine triphosphatase
✦ Results in shortening of action potential and contributes to shortening of atrial and ventricular refractoriness
✦ Enhances vagal tone and slows conduction through SA and AV nodes

ECG characteristics

✦ *Rate*—atrial and ventricular rates decreased
✦ *PR interval*—shortened
✦ *T wave*—decreased
✦ *ST segment*—shortened and depressed
✦ *QT interval*—shortened due to shortened ST segment
✦ Digoxin has narrow window of therapeutic effectiveness; at toxic levels, may cause numerous arrhythmias

DIGOXIN

Digoxin, the most commonly used cardiac glycoside, works by inhibiting the enzyme adenosine triphosphatase. This enzyme is found in the plasma membrane and acts as a pump to exchange sodium ions for potassium ions. Inhibition of sodium-potassium–activated adenosine triphosphatase results in enhanced movement of calcium from the extracellular space to the intracellular space, thereby strengthening myocardial contractions.

The effects of digoxin on the electrical properties of the heart include direct and autonomic effects. Direct effects result in shortening of the action potential, which contributes to the shortening of atrial and ventricular refractoriness. Autonomic effects involve the sympathetic and parasympathetic systems. Vagal tone is enhanced, and conduction through the sinoatrial (SA) and atrioventricular (AV) nodes is slowed. The drug also exerts an antiarrhythmic effect.

Digoxin is indicated in the treatment of heart failure, paroxysmal supraventricular tachycardia, atrial fibrillation, and atrial flutter.

ECG CHARACTERISTICS

When a patient is taking digoxin, you may see these ECG changes:
✦ *Rate:* Atrial and ventricular rates are decreased.
✦ *PR interval:* Shortened.
✦ *T wave:* Decreased.

ECG effects of digoxin

Digoxin affects the cardiac cycle in various ways and may lead to the ECG changes shown here.

ECG characteristics of digoxin:

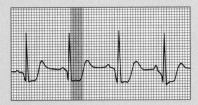

✦ *ST segment:* gradual sloping, causing ST-segment depression in the opposite direction of the QRS deflection (shaded area)

✦ *P wave:* may be notched

◆ *ST segment:* Shortened and depressed. Sagging (scooping or sloping) of the segment is characteristic.

◆ *QT interval:* Shortened due to the shortened ST segment.

◆ Digoxin has a very narrow window of therapeutic effectiveness and, at toxic levels, may cause numerous arrhythmias, including paroxysmal atrial tachycardia with block, AV block, atrial and junctional tachyarrhythmias, and ventricular arrhythmias. (See *ECG effects of digoxin.*)

Nonpharmacologic treatment

Nonpharmacologic interventions produce distinctive electrocardiogram (ECG) tracings. These interventions include various types of pacemakers, implantable cardioverter defibrillators, radiofrequency ablation, and ventricular assist devices.

PACEMAKERS

A pacemaker is an artificial device that electrically stimulates the myocardium to depolarize, initiating mechanical contractions. It works by generating an impulse from a power source and transmitting that impulse to the heart muscle. The impulse flows throughout the heart and causes the heart muscle to depolarize.

A pacemaker may be used when a patient has an arrhythmia, such as certain bradyarrhythmias and tachyarrhythmias, sick sinus syndrome (SSS), or an atrioventricular (AV) block. The device may be used as a temporary measure or a permanent one, depending on the patient's condition. Pacemakers are typically necessary following myocardial infarction or cardiac surgery.

This section examines how pacemakers work, ECG characteristics, types of pacemakers, synchronous and asynchronous pacing, biventricular pacemakers, description codes, pacing modes, assessment of pacemaker function, troubleshooting a pacemaker, interventions, and patient teaching.

Pacemakers
+ Stimulate myocardium to depolarize, initiating mechanical contractions
+ Used for certain bradyarrhythmias and tachyarrhythmias, SSS, or AV block
+ Can be temporary or permanent

How pacemakers work

- Three components: pulse generator, pacing leads, and one or more electrodes at distal ends of leadwires
- Electrical stimulus from pulse generator moves through pacing leads to electrode tips
- Electrodes send data about impulses in myocardium back to pulse generator
- Pulse generator senses heart's electrical activity, responding accordingly
- Unipolar lead system more sensitive to heart's intrinsic electrical activity

HOW PACEMAKERS WORK

A typical pacemaker has three main components: a pulse generator, pacing leads or wires, and one or more electrodes at the distal ends of leadwires. The pulse generator contains the pacemaker's power source and circuitry. It creates an electrical impulse that moves through the pacing leads to the electrodes, transmitting that impulse to the heart muscle and causing the heart to depolarize. The lithium battery in a permanent or implanted pacemaker serves as its power source and lasts between 5 and 10 years. A microchip in the device guides heart pacing.

A temporary pacemaker, which isn't implanted, is about the size of a small radio or telemetry box and is powered by alkaline batteries. These units also contain a microchip and are programmed by a touch pad or dials.

An electrical stimulus from the pulse generator moves through wires, or pacing leads, to the electrode tips. The leads for a pacemaker, designed to stimulate a single heart chamber, are placed in either the atrium or the ventricle. For dual-chamber, or AV, pacing, the leads are placed in both chambers, usually on the right side of the heart. (See *Pacing leads.*)

The electrodes — one on a unipolar lead or two on a bipolar lead — send information about electrical impulses in the myocardium back to the pulse generator. The pulse generator senses the heart's electrical activity and responds according to how it was programmed.

Pacing leads

Pacing leads have either one electrode (unipolar) or two (bipolar). These illustrations show the difference between the two leads.

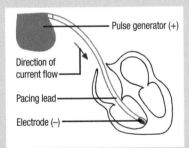

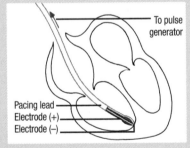

UNIPOLAR LEAD
In a unipolar system, electric current moves from the pulse generator through the leadwire to the negative pole. From there, it stimulates the heart and returns to the pulse generator's metal surface (the positive pole) to complete the circuit.

BIPOLAR LEAD
In a bipolar system, current flows from the pulse generator through the leadwire to the negative pole at the tip. At that point, it stimulates the heart and then flows back to the positive pole to complete the circuit.

A unipolar lead system is more sensitive to the heart's intrinsic electrical activity than a bipolar system. A bipolar system isn't as easily affected by electrical activity, such as skeletal muscle contraction or magnetic fields, originating outside the heart and the generator. A bipolar system is more difficult to implant, however.

ECG CHARACTERISTICS

The most prominent characteristic of a pacemaker on an ECG is the pacemaker spike. (See *Pacemaker spikes.*) It occurs when the pacemaker sends an electrical impulse to the heart muscle. The impulse appears as a vertical line, or spike. The collective group of spikes on an ECG is called pacemaker artifact.

Depending on the electrode's position, the spike appears in different locations on the waveform:

✦ When the pacemaker stimulates the atria, the spike is followed by a P wave and the patient's baseline QRS complex and T wave. This series of waveforms represents successful pacing, or capture, of the myocardium. The P wave appears different from the patient's normal P wave.

✦ When the ventricles are stimulated by a pacemaker, the spike is followed by a QRS complex and a T wave. The QRS complex appears wider than the patient's own QRS complex because of how the pacemaker depolarizes the ventricles.

✦ When the pacemaker stimulates both the atria and ventricles, the spike is followed by a P wave, then a spike, and then a QRS complex. Be aware that the type of pacemaker used and the patient's condition may affect whether every beat is paced.

ECG characteristics

✦ Most prominent characteristic is pacemaker spike (when pacemaker sends electrical impulse to heart muscle)
✦ If pacemaker stimulates atria, spike followed by P wave and baseline QRS complex and T wave
✦ If pacemaker stimulates ventricles, spike followed by QRS complex and T wave
✦ If pacemaker stimulates atria and ventricles, spike followed by P wave, spike, and then QRS complex

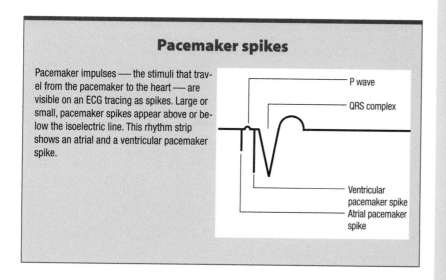

Pacemaker spikes

Pacemaker impulses — the stimuli that travel from the pacemaker to the heart — are visible on an ECG tracing as spikes. Large or small, pacemaker spikes appear above or below the isoelectric line. This rhythm strip shows an atrial and a ventricular pacemaker spike.

P wave
QRS complex
Ventricular pacemaker spike
Atrial pacemaker spike

+ Treat chronic heart conditions
+ Surgically implanted, with leads placed transvenously in appropriate chambers
+ Generator implanted in pocket made from subcutaneous tissue

PERMANENT PACEMAKERS

A permanent pacemaker is used to treat chronic heart conditions such as AV block. It's surgically implanted, usually under local anesthesia. The leads are placed transvenously, positioned in the appropriate chambers, and then anchored to the endocardium. (See *Placing a permanent pacemaker.*)

The generator is then implanted in a pocket made from subcutaneous tissue. The pocket is usually constructed under the clavicle. Most permanent pacemakers are programmed before implantation. The programming sets the conditions under which the pacemaker functions and can be adjusted externally if necessary.

BIVENTRICULAR PACEMAKERS

Biventricular pacing, also referred to as *cardiac resynchronization therapy,* is used to treat patients with moderate and severe heart failure who have left

---

Placing a permanent pacemaker

Implanting a pacemaker is a simple surgical procedure performed with local anesthesia and conscious sedation. To implant an endocardial pacemaker, the surgeon usually selects a transvenous route and begins lead placement by inserting a catheter percutaneously or by venous cutdown. Then, using fluoroscopic guidance, the surgeon threads the catheter through the vein until the tip reaches the endocardium.

LEAD PLACEMENT
For lead placement in the atrium, the tip must lodge in the right atrium or coronary sinus, as shown here. For placement in the ventricle, it must lodge in the right ventricular apex in one of the interior muscular ridges, or trabeculae.

IMPLANTING THE GENERATOR
When the lead is in proper position, the surgeon secures the pulse generator in a subcutaneous pocket of tissue just below the patient's clavicle. Changing the generator's battery or microchip circuitry requires only a shallow incision over the site and a quick exchange of components.

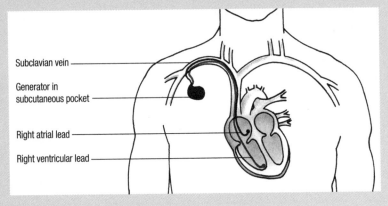

Subclavian vein

Generator in subcutaneous pocket

Right atrial lead

Right ventricular lead

ventricular dyssynchrony. These patients have intraventricular conduction defects, which result in uncoordinated contraction of the right and left ventricles and a wide QRS complex on an ECG. Left ventricular dyssynchrony has been associated with worsening heart failure and increased morbidity and mortality.

Under normal conditions, the right and left ventricles contract simultaneously to pump blood to the lungs and body, respectively. However, in heart failure, the damaged ventricles can't pump as forcefully and the amount of blood ejected with each contraction is reduced. If the ventricular conduction pathways are also damaged, electrical impulses reach the ventricles at different times, producing asynchronous contractions (intraventricular conduction defect), which further reduces the amount of blood that the heart pumps, worsening the patient's symptoms.

To compensate for this reduced cardiac output, the sympathetic nervous system releases neurohormones, such as aldosterone, norepinephrine, and vasopressin, to boost the amount of blood ejected with each contraction. The resultant tachycardia and vasoconstriction increase the heart's demand for oxygen, reduce diastolic filling time, promote sodium and water retention, and increase the pressure that the heart must pump against.

To coordinate ventricular contractions and improve hemodynamic status, biventricular pacemakers use three leads—one in the right atrium and one in each ventricle. Both ventricles are paced at the same time, causing them to contract simultaneously, thereby increasing cardiac output.

Unlike traditional lead placement, the electrode tip for the left ventricle is placed in the coronary sinus to a branch of the inferior cardiac vein. Because this electrode tip isn't anchored in place, lead displacement may occur. (See *Biventricular lead placement,* page 172.)

Biventricular pacing produces an immediate improvement in the patient's symptoms and activity tolerance. Moreover, biventricular pacing improves left ventricular remodeling and diastolic function and reduces sympathetic stimulation. As a result, in many patients the progression of heart failure is slowed and quality of life is improved.

Who's a candidate?
Not all patients with heart failure benefit from biventricular pacing. Candidates should have both systolic heart failure and ventricular dyssynchrony along with the following characteristics:
+ symptom-producing heart failure despite maximal medical therapy
+ moderate to severe heart failure (New York Heart Association class III or IV)
+ QRS complex greater than 0.13 second
+ left ventricular ejection fraction of 35% or less.

Biventricular pacemakers
+ Treat moderate and severe heart failure, with left ventricular dyssynchrony
+ Three leads coordinate ventricular contractions: one in right atrium and one in each ventricle
+ Ventricles paced simultaneously, increasing output
+ Produces immediate improvement in symptoms and activity tolerance
+ Improves left ventricular remodeling and diastolic function and reduces sympathetic stimulation

Who's a candidate?
Systolic heart failure and ventricular dyssynchrony are present along with:
+ symptom-producing heart failure, despite maximal medical therapy
+ moderate to severe heart failure
+ QRS complex > 0.13 second
+ left ventricular ejection fraction of 35% or less

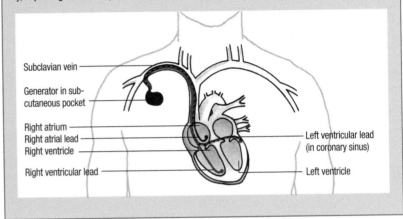

Biventricular lead placement

The biventricular pacemaker uses three leads: one to pace the right atrium, one to pace the right ventricle, and one to pace the left ventricle. The left ventricular lead is placed in the coronary sinus. Both ventricles are paced at the same time, causing them to contract simultaneously, improving cardiac output.

Pacemaker description codes

✦ Five-letter coding system (though use of three is more common)

Pacing modes

✦ Indicates functions and includes AAI, VVI, DVI, and DDD

AAI mode

✦ Single-chambered pacemaker paces and senses atria
✦ When pacemaker senses intrinsic atrial activity, it inhibits pacing and resets itself

PACEMAKER DESCRIPTION CODES

The capabilities of permanent pacemakers are described by a five-letter coding system, though three letters are more commonly used. (See *Pacemaker coding systems.*)

PACING MODES

A pacemaker's mode indicates its functions. Several different modes may be used during pacing, and they may not mimic the normal cardiac cycle. A three-letter code, rather than a five-letter code, is typically used to describe pacemaker function. Modes include AAI, VVI, DVI, and DDD. (See *AAI and VVI pacemakers,* page 174.)

AAI mode

The AAI, or atrial demand, pacemaker is a single-chambered pacemaker that paces and senses the atria. When the pacemaker senses intrinsic atrial activity, it inhibits pacing and resets itself. Only the atria are paced.

Because AAI pacemakers require a functioning AV node and intact conduction system, they aren't used in AV block. An AAI pacemaker may be used in patients with sinus bradycardia, which may occur after cardiac surgery, or with SSS, as long as the AV node and His-Purkinje system aren't diseased.

Pacemaker coding systems

The capabilities of permanent pacemakers can be described by a five-letter coding system. Typically, only the first three letters are used.

FIRST LETTER
The first letter identifies which heart chambers are paced:
+ V = Ventricle
+ A = Atrium
+ D = Dual — ventricle and atrium
+ 0 = None.

SECOND LETTER
The second letter signifies the heart chamber where the pacemaker senses intrinsic activity:
+ V = Ventricle
+ A = Atrium
+ D = Dual
+ 0 = None.

THIRD LETTER
The third letter indicates the pacemaker's mode of response to the intrinsic electrical activity it senses in the atrium or ventricle:
+ T = Triggers pacing
+ I = Inhibits pacing
+ D = Dual — can trigger or inhibit depending on the mode and where intrinsic activity occurs
+ 0 = None — doesn't change mode in response to sensed activity.

FOURTH LETTER
The fourth letter describes the degree of programmability and the presence or absence of an adaptive rate response:
+ P = Basic functions programmable
+ M = Multiprogrammable parameters
+ C = Communicating functions such as telemetry
+ R = Rate responsiveness — rate adjusts to fit the patient's metabolic needs and achieve normal hemodynamic status
+ 0 = None.

FIFTH LETTER
The fifth letter denotes the pacemaker's response to a tachyarrhythmia:
+ P = Pacing ability — the pacemaker's rapid burst paces the heart at a rate above its intrinsic rate to override the tachycardia source
+ S = Shock — an implantable cardioverter-defibrillator identifies ventricular tachycardia and delivers a shock to stop the arrhythmia
+ D = Dual ability to shock and pace
+ 0 = None.

VVI mode

The VVI, or ventricular demand, pacemaker paces and senses the ventricles. When it senses intrinsic ventricular activity, it inhibits pacing.

This single-chambered pacemaker benefits patients with complete heart block and those needing intermittent pacing. Because it doesn't affect atrial activity, it's used for patients who don't need an atrial kick — the extra 15% to 30% of cardiac output that comes from atrial contraction.

If a patient has spontaneous atrial activity, a VVI pacemaker won't synchronize the ventricular activity with it, so tricuspid and mitral insufficiency may develop. Sedentary patients may receive this pacemaker, but it won't adjust its rate for more active patients.

VVI mode
+ Paces and senses ventricles
+ When pacemaker senses intrinsic ventricular activity, it inhibits pacing

AAI and VVI pacemakers

AAI and VVI pacemakers are single-chamber pacemakers. The electrode is placed in the atrium for an AAI pacemaker, in the ventricle for a VVI pacemaker. These rhythm strips show how each pacemaker works.

AAI PACEMAKER

An AAI pacemaker senses and paces only the atria. As shown in the shaded area below, a P wave follows each atrial spike (atrial depolarization). The QRS complexes reflect the heart's own conduction.

This pacemaker requires a functioning atrioventricular node and intact conduction system. It may be used in patients who have symptom-producing sinus bradycardia or sick sinus syndrome.

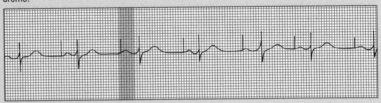

VVI PACEMAKER

A VVI pacemaker senses and paces the ventricles. When each spike is followed by a QRS complex (depolarization), as shown here, the rhythm is said to reflect 100% capture.

This pacemaker may be used in patients who have chronic atrial fibrillation with slow ventricular response and those who need infrequent pacing.

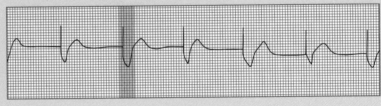

DVI mode

- ✦ Dual-chambered pacemaker paces atria and ventricles
- ✦ Senses ventricles' intrinsic activity only, inhibiting ventricular pacing

Two types of DVI pacemakers
- ✦ *Committed*—generates impulse even with spontaneous ventricular depolarization
- ✦ *Noncommitted*—only inhibited if spontaneous depolarization occurs

DVI mode

The DVI, or AV sequential, pacemaker paces the atria and ventricles. (See *DVI pacemakers.*) This dual-chambered pacemaker senses only the ventricles' intrinsic activity, inhibiting ventricular pacing.

Two types of DVI pacemakers may be used, a committed DVI and a noncommitted DVI pacemaker. The committed DVI pacemaker doesn't sense intrinsic activity during the AV interval—the time between an atrial and ventricular spike. It generates an impulse even with spontaneous ventricular depolarization. The noncommitted DVI pacemaker, on the other hand, is inhibited if a spontaneous depolarization occurs.

The DVI pacemaker helps patients with AV block or SSS who have a diseased His-Purkinje conduction system. It provides the benefits of AV synchrony and atrial kick, thus improving cardiac output. However, it can't vary

---

DVI pacemakers

A committed DVI pacemaker (also known as an *atrioventricular (AV) sequential pacemaker*) senses ventricular activity and paces the atria and ventricles, firing despite the intrinsic QRS complex. The rhythm strip shown here shows the effects of a committed DVI pacemaker. Notice that in two of the complexes, shown with shaded areas, the pacemaker didn't sense the intrinsic QRS complex because the complex occurred during the AV interval, when the pacemaker was already committed to fire.

With a noncommitted DVI pacemaker, spikes wouldn't appear after the QRS complex because the stimulus to pace the ventricles would be inhibited.

ECG characteristics of committed DVI pacemaker:

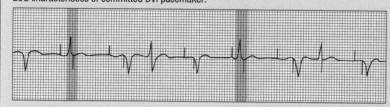

✦ Ventricular pacemaker: fires despite the intrinsic QRS complex

---

the atrial rate and isn't helpful in atrial fibrillation because it can't capture the atria. In addition, it may needlessly fire or inhibit its own pacing.

DDD mode

A DDD, or universal, pacemaker is used with severe AV block. (See *DDD pacemakers*, page 176.) However, because the pacemaker possesses so many capabilities, it may be hard to troubleshoot problems.

Advantages of the DDD pacemaker include its:

✦ versatility
✦ programmability
✦ ability to change modes automatically
✦ ability to mimic the normal physiologic cardiac cycle, maintaining AV synchrony
✦ ability to sense and pace the atria and ventricles at the same time according to the intrinsic atrial rate and maximal rate limit.

Unlike other pacemakers, the DDD pacemaker is set with a rate range, rather than a single critical rate. It senses atrial activity and ensures that the ventricles respond to each atrial stimulation, thereby maintaining normal AV synchrony.

The DDD pacemaker fires when the ventricle doesn't respond on its own, and it paces the atria when the atrial rate falls below the lower set rate. In a patient with a high atrial rate, a safety mechanism allows the pacemaker to

DDD mode
✦ Used with severe AV block; set with a rate range
✦ Senses atrial activity and ensures that ventricles respond to each atrial stimulation
✦ Fires when ventricle doesn't respond on its own and paces atria when rate falls below lower set rate
✦ With high atrial rate, safety mechanism allows pacemaker to follow intrinsic atrial rate only to preset upper limit

DDD pacemakers

When evaluating the rhythm strip of a patient with a DDD pacemaker, keep several points in mind.
+ If the patient has an adequate intrinsic rhythm, the pacemaker won't fire; it doesn't need to.
+ If you see an intrinsic P wave followed by a ventricular pacemaker spike, the pacemaker is tracking the atrial rate and assuring a ventricular response.
+ If you see a pacemaker spike before a P wave, followed by an intrinsic ventricular QRS complex, the atrial rate is falling below the lower rate limit, causing the atrial channel to fire. Normal conduction to the ventricles follows.
+ If you see a pacemaker spike before a P wave and before the QRS complex, no intrinsic activity is taking place in either the atria or ventricles.

In this rhythm strip, complexes 1, 2, 4, and 7 show the atrial-synchronous mode, set at a rate of 70. The patient has an intrinsic P wave, so the pacemaker only ensures that the ventricles respond. Complexes 3, 5, 8, 10, and 12 are intrinsic ventricular depolarizations. The pacemaker senses them and doesn't fire. In complexes 6, 9, and 11, the pacemaker is pacing the atria and ventricles in sequence. In complex 13, only the atria are paced; the ventricles respond on their own.

ECG characteristics of DDD pacemakers:

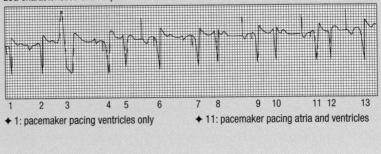

+ 1: pacemaker pacing ventricles only   + 11: pacemaker pacing atria and ventricles

follow the intrinsic atrial rate only to a preset upper limit. That limit is usually set at about 130 beats/minute and helps to prevent the ventricles from responding to atrial tachycardia or atrial flutter.

TEMPORARY PACEMAKERS

A temporary pacemaker is commonly inserted in an emergency. The patient may show signs of decreased cardiac output, such as hypotension or syncope. The temporary pacemaker supports the patient until the condition resolves.

A temporary pacemaker can also serve as a bridge until a permanent pacemaker is inserted. These pacemakers are used for patients with high-grade heart block, bradycardia, or low cardiac output. Several types of temporary pacemakers are available, including transvenous, epicardial, transcutaneous, and transthoracic.

Transvenous pacemakers

Physicians usually use the transvenous approach — inserting the pacemaker through a vein, such as the subclavian or internal jugular vein — when inserting a temporary pacemaker. The transvenous pacemaker is probably the most common and reliable type of temporary pacemaker. It's usually inserted at the bedside or in a fluoroscopy suite. The leadwires are advanced through a catheter into the right ventricle or atrium and then connected to the pulse generator.

Epicardial pacemakers

Epicardial pacemakers are commonly used for patients undergoing cardiac surgery. The tips of the leadwires are attached to the heart's surface and then the wires are brought through the chest wall, below the incision. They're then attached to the pulse generator. The leadwires are usually removed several days after surgery or when the patient no longer requires them.

Transcutaneous pacemakers

Use of an external or transcutaneous pacemaker has become commonplace in the past several years. In this noninvasive method, one electrode is placed on the patient's anterior chest wall to the right of the upper sternum below the clavicle and a second electrode is applied to his back (anterior-posterior electrodes). One may also be placed to the left of the left nipple with the center of the electrode in the midaxillary line (also called the anterior-apex position). An external pulse generator then emits pacing impulses that travel through the skin to the heart muscle. Transcutaneous pacing is built into many defibrillators for use in emergencies. In this case, the electrodes are built into the same pads used for defibrillation.

Transcutaneous pacing is a quick, effective method of pacing heart rhythm and is commonly used in emergencies until a transvenous pacemaker can be inserted. However, some patients may not be able to tolerate the irritating sensations produced from prolonged pacing at the levels needed to pace the heart externally. If hemodynamically stable, these patients may require sedation.

Transvenous pacemakers

+ Most common and reliable type, inserted at bedside or in fluoroscopy suite
+ Inserted through subclavian or internal jugular vein

Epicardial pacemakers

+ Commonly used when undergoing cardiac surgery
+ Leadwire tips attached to heart's surface then brought through chest wall below incision

Transcutaneous pacemakers

+ Commonly used in emergencies until insertion of transvenous pacemaker
+ One electrode placed on anterior chest wall; second electrode applied to back
+ One may also be placed to left of left nipple with center of electrode in midaxillary line

Transthoracic pacemakers

+ Only used as last resort; insertion of needle into right ventricle, using subxiphoid approach

Temporary pacemaker settings

+ Rate control regulates number of impulses generated in 1 minute; measured in ppm
+ Energy output measured in mA; represents stimulation threshold
+ Sensitivity measured in millivolts; senses heart's normal activity

Synchronous and asynchronous pacing

Synchronous (demand)
+ Initiates electrical impulses only when heart's intrinsic rate falls below preset rate

Asynchronous (fixed)
+ Initiates electrical impulses at preset rate regardless of intrinsic activity or heart rate

Transthoracic pacemakers

A transthoracic pacemaker is a type of temporary ventricular pacemaker only used during cardiac emergencies as a last resort. Transthoracic pacing requires insertion of a long needle into the right ventricle, using a subxiphoid approach. A pacing wire is then guided directly into the endocardium.

TEMPORARY PACEMAKER SETTINGS

A temporary pacemaker has several types of settings on the pulse generator. The rate control regulates how many impulses are generated in 1 minute and is measured in pulses per minute (ppm). The rate is usually set at 60 to 80 ppm. (See *Temporary pulse generator.*) The pacemaker fires if the patient's heart rate falls below the preset rate. The rate may be set higher if the patient has a tachyarrhythmia being treated with overdrive pacing.

A pacemaker's energy output is measured in milliamperes (mA), a measurement that represents the stimulation threshold, or how much energy is required to stimulate the cardiac muscle to depolarize. The stimulation threshold is sometimes referred to as *energy required for capture.*

You can also program the pacemaker's sensitivity, measured in millivolts. Most pacemakers allow the heart to function naturally and assist only when necessary. The sensing threshold allows the pacemaker to do this by sensing the heart's normal activity.

SYNCHRONOUS AND ASYNCHRONOUS PACING

Pacemakers can be classified according to sensitivity. In synchronous, or demand, pacing, the pacemaker initiates electrical impulses only when the heart's intrinsic heart rate falls below the preset rate of the pacemaker. In asynchronous, or fixed, pacing, the pacemaker constantly initiates electrical impulses at a preset rate without regard to the patient's intrinsic electrical activity or heart rate. This type of pacemaker is rarely used.

ASSESSING PACEMAKER FUNCTION

After a pacemaker has been implanted, its function should be assessed. First, determine the pacemaker's mode and settings. If the patient had a permanent pacemaker implanted before admission, ask whether the wallet card from the manufacturer notes the mode and settings.

If the pacemaker was recently implanted, check the patient's medical record for information about the pacemaker settings because this will help prevent misinterpretation of the ECG tracing. For instance, if the tracing has ventricular spikes but no atrial pacing spikes, you might assume that it's a VVI pacemaker when it's a DVI pacemaker that has lost its atrial output.

Temporary pulse generator

The settings on a temporary pulse generator may be changed in several ways to meet the patient's specific needs. The illustration below shows a single-chamber temporary pulse generator and brief descriptions of its various parts.

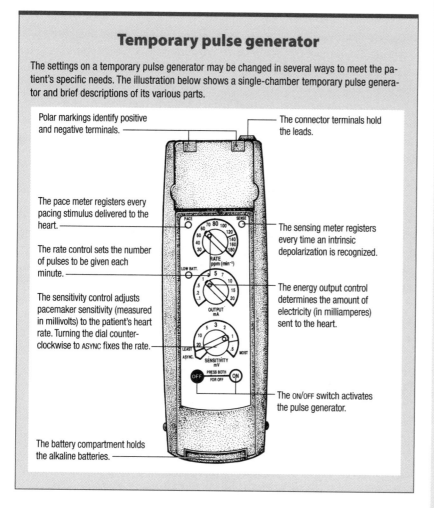

Polar markings identify positive and negative terminals.

The connector terminals hold the leads.

The pace meter registers every pacing stimulus delivered to the heart.

The rate control sets the number of pulses to be given each minute.

The sensitivity control adjusts pacemaker sensitivity (measured in millivolts) to the patient's heart rate. Turning the dial counter-clockwise to ASYNC fixes the rate.

The sensing meter registers every time an intrinsic depolarization is recognized.

The energy output control determines the amount of electricity (in milliamperes) sent to the heart.

The ON/OFF switch activates the pulse generator.

The battery compartment holds the alkaline batteries.

Next, review the patient's 12-lead ECG. If it isn't available, examine lead V_1 or MCL_1 instead.

Select a monitoring lead that clearly shows the pacemaker spikes. Make sure the lead you select doesn't cause the cardiac monitor to misinterpret a spike for a QRS complex and double-count the heart rate. This may cause the alarm to sound, falsely signaling a high heart rate.

When looking at an ECG tracing for a patient with a pacemaker, consider the pacemaker mode, and then interpret the paced rhythm. Does it correlate with what you know about the pacemaker?

Look for information that tells you which chamber is paced. Is there capture? Is there a P wave or QRS complex after each atrial or ventricular spike? Or do the P waves and QRS complexes stem from intrinsic electrical activity?

Look for information about the pacemaker's sensing ability. If intrinsic atrial or ventricular activity is present, what's the pacemaker's response?

Assessing pacemaker function

- ✦ Determine mode and settings
- ✦ Ask whether wallet card from manufacturer notes mode and settings (with permanent)
- ✦ Review 12-lead ECG
- ✦ Select monitoring lead that clearly shows spikes
- ✦ Look for information that shows which chamber is paced
- ✦ Determine sensing ability and rate

Look at the rate. What's the pacing rate per minute? Is it appropriate given the pacemaker settings? Although you can determine the rate quickly by counting the number of complexes in a 6-second ECG strip, a more accurate method is to count the number of small boxes between complexes and divide this into 1,500.

Knowing your patient's medical history and whether a pacemaker has been implanted will also help you to determine whether your patient is experiencing ventricular ectopy or paced activity on the ECG. (See *Distinguishing intermittent ventricular pacing from PVCs.*)

TROUBLESHOOTING PACEMAKER PROBLEMS

A malfunctioning pacemaker can lead to arrhythmias, hypotension, syncope, and other signs and symptoms of decreased cardiac output. (See *Recognizing a malfunctioning pacemaker,* pages 182 and 183.) Common problems with pacemakers that can lead to low cardiac output and loss of AV synchrony include:

✦ failure to capture
✦ failure to pace
✦ undersensing
✦ oversensing.

Failure to capture

Failure to capture appears on an ECG as a pacemaker spike without the appropriate atrial or ventricular response—a spike without a complex. Think of failure to capture as the pacemaker's inability to stimulate the chamber.

Causes of failure to capture include acidosis, electrolyte imbalances, fibrosis, incorrect leadwire position, a low mA or output setting, depletion of the battery, a broken or cracked leadwire, or perforation of the leadwire through the myocardium.

Failure to pace

Failure to pace is indicated by no pacemaker activity on an ECG when pacemaker activity is appropriately expected. This problem may be caused by battery or circuit failure, cracked or broken leads, or interference between atrial and ventricular sensing in a dual-chambered pacemaker. Failure to pace can lead to asystole.

Undersensing

Undersensing is indicated by a pacemaker spike when intrinsic cardiac activity is present. In asynchronous pacemakers that have codes, such as VOO or DOO, undersensing is a programming limitation.

When undersensing occurs in synchronous pacemakers, pacing spikes occur on the ECG where they shouldn't. Although they may appear in any part

---

Failure to capture

✦ Pacemaker spike without appropriate atrial or ventricular response

Causes
✦ Acidosis
✦ Electrolyte imbalances
✦ Fibrosis
✦ Incorrect leadwire position
✦ Low mA or output setting
✦ Depletion of battery
✦ Broken or cracked leadwire
✦ Perforation of leadwire through myocardium

Failure to pace

✦ Absence of pacemaker activity when activity is expected

Causes
✦ Battery or circuit failure
✦ Cracked or broken leads
✦ Interference between atrial and ventricular sensing

12-lead ECG

One of the most valuable and frequently used diagnostic tools, an electrocardiogram (ECG) measures the heart's electrical activity as waveforms. Impulses moving through the heart's conduction system create electric currents that can be monitored on the body's surface. Electrodes attached to the skin (as shown below) can detect these electric currents and transmit them to an instrument that produces a record (the ECG strip) of cardiac activity.

ECGs can be used to identify myocardial ischemia, injury, and infarction; rhythm and conduction disturbances; chamber enlargement; electrolyte imbalances; and drug toxicity.

ECG ELECTRODE PLACEMENT

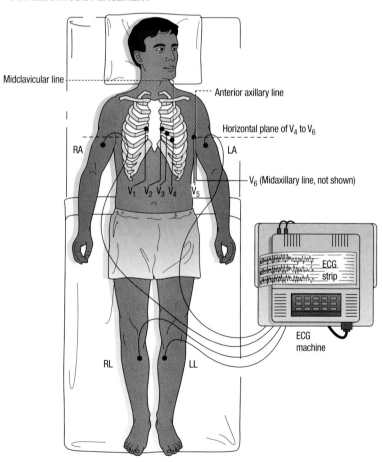

Myocardial infarction

Remember the three I's of myocardial infarction: ischemia, injury, and infarction. These three pathologic changes are related but produce different effects on the myocardium.

During the ischemic phase, the patient may experience angina, a result of deficient delivery of blood and oxygen to the myocardium.

If the blood and oxygen supply isn't improved and ischemia continues, injury to the myocardium is inevitable. Eventually, infarction or tissue necrosis causes irreversible damage.

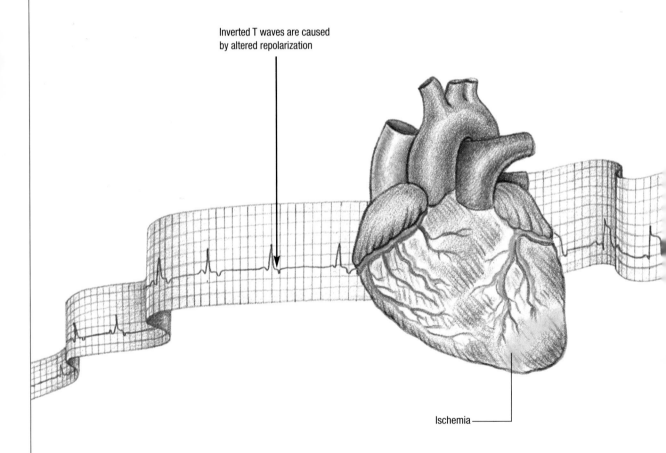

Inverted T waves are caused by altered repolarization

Ischemia

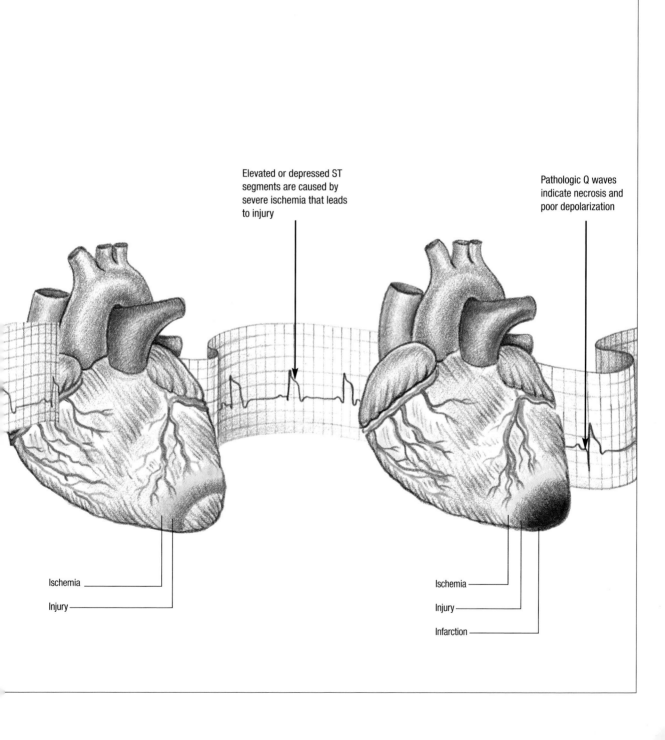

Elevated or depressed ST segments are caused by severe ischemia that leads to injury

Pathologic Q waves indicate necrosis and poor depolarization

Ischemia

Injury

Ischemia

Injury

Infarction

Localizing myocardial ischemia, injury, or infarction

Identifying the location of myocardial ischemia, injury, or infarction is critical in determining appropriate treatment and predicting possible complications. Characteristic ECG changes are localized to the leads overlying the infarction site. The illustration below highlights the leads that identify areas of damage in specific walls of the heart.

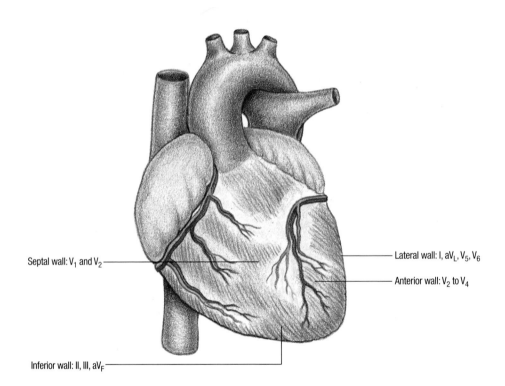

Septal wall: V_1 and V_2

Lateral wall: I, aV_L, V_5, V_6

Anterior wall: V_2 to V_4

Inferior wall: II, III, aV_F

LOOK-ALIKES

Distinguishing intermittent ventricular pacing from PVCs

Knowing whether your patient has an artificial pacemaker will help you avoid mistaking a ventricular paced beat for a premature ventricular contraction (PVC). If your facility uses a monitoring system that eliminates artifact, make sure the monitor is set up correctly for a patient with a pacemaker. Otherwise, the pacemaker spikes may be eliminated as well.

If your patient has intermittent ventricular pacing, the paced ventricular complex will have a pacemaker spike preceding it, as shown in the shaded area of the top ECG strip. You may need to look in different leads for a bipolar pacemaker spike because it's small and may be difficult to see. What's more, the paced ventricular complex of a properly functioning pacemaker won't occur early or prematurely, it will occur only when the patient's own ventricular rate falls below the rate set for the pacemaker.

If your patient is having PVCs, they'll occur prematurely and won't have pacemaker spikes preceding them. Examples are shown in the shaded areas of the bottom ECG strip.

INTERMITTENT VENTRICULAR PACING

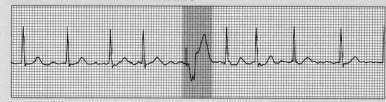

PVCs

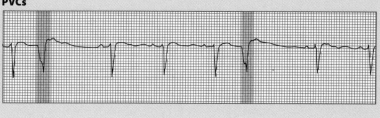

of the cardiac cycle, the spikes are especially dangerous if they fall on the T wave, where they can cause ventricular tachycardia or ventricular fibrillation.

In synchronous pacemakers, undersensing may be caused by electrolyte imbalances, disconnection or dislodgment of a lead, improper lead placement, increased sensing threshold from edema or fibrosis at the electrode tip, drug interactions, or a depleted or dead pacemaker battery.

Undersensing

✦ Pacemaker spike when intrinsic cardiac activity is present
✦ Spikes dangerous if they fall on T wave (ventricular tachycardia or fibrillation may develop)

Causes

✦ Electrolyte imbalances
✦ Disconnection or dislodgement of lead
✦ Improper lead placement
✦ Increased sensing threshold from edema or fibrosis at electrode tip
✦ Drug interactions
✦ Depleted or dead battery

Recognizing a malfunctioning pacemaker

Occasionally, pacemakers fail to function properly. When this happens, you'll need to take immediate action to correct the problem. The rhythm strips below show examples of problems that can occur with a temporary pacemaker.

FAILURE TO CAPTURE

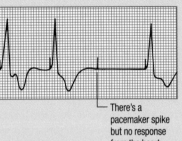

There's a pacemaker spike but no response from the heart.

+ ECG shows a pacemaker spike without the appropriate atrial or ventricular response (spike without a complex), as shown at right.
+ Patient may be asymptomatic or have signs of decreased cardiac output.
+ Pacemaker can't stimulate the chamber.
+ Problem may be caused by increased pacing thresholds related to certain situations:
  – Metabolic or electrolyte imbalance
  – Antiarrhythmics
  – Fibrosis or edema at electrode tip
+ Problem may be caused by lead malfunction:
  – Dislodged lead
  – Broken or damaged lead
  – Perforation of myocardium by lead
  – Loose connection between lead and pulse generator
+ Related interventions may solve the problem:
  – Treat metabolic disturbance.
  – Replace damaged lead.
  – Change pulse generator battery.
  – Slowly increase output setting until capture occurs.
  – A chest X-ray may be needed to determine electrode placement.

FAILURE TO PACE

+ ECG shows no pacemaker activity when pacemaker activity should be evident, as shown at right.
+ Magnet application yields no response. (It should cause asynchronous pacing.)
+ Problem has several common causes:
  – Depleted battery
  – Circuit failure
  – Lead malfunction
  – Inappropriate programming of sensing function
  – Electromagnetic interference

A pacemaker spike should appear here but doesn't.

+ Failure to pace can lead to asystole or a severe decrease in cardiac output in pacemaker-dependent patients.
+ If you think a pacemaker is failing to pace, a temporary pacemaker (transcutaneous or transvenous) should be used to prevent asystole.
+ Related interventions may solve the problem:
  – Replace pulse generator battery.
  – Replace pulse generator unit.
  – Adjust sensitivity setting.
  – Remove source of electromagnetic interference.

Recognizing a malfunctioning pacemaker (continued)

FAILURE TO SENSE INTRINSIC BEATS (UNDERSENSING)

◆ ECG may show pacing spikes anywhere in the cycle, as shown at right.
◆ A pacemaker spike may appear where intrinsic cardiac activity is present.
◆ Patient may report feeling palpitations or skipped beats.
◆ Spikes are especially dangerous if they fall on the T wave because ventricular tachycardia or fibrillation may result.
◆ Problem has several common causes:
  – Battery failure
  – Fracture of pacing leadwire
  – Displacement of electrode tip
  – "Cross-talk" between atrial and ventricular channels
  – Electromagnetic interference mistaken for intrinsic signals
◆ Related interventions may solve the problem:
  – Replace the pulse generator battery.
  – Replace the leadwires.
  – Adjust the sensitivity setting.

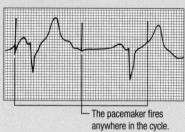

The pacemaker fires anywhere in the cycle.

Oversensing

If the pacemaker is too sensitive, it can misinterpret muscle movements or other events in the cardiac cycle as intrinsic cardiac electrical activity. Pacing won't occur when it's needed, and the heart rate and AV synchrony won't be maintained.

INTERVENTIONS

Make sure you're familiar with different types of pacemakers and how they function, so you'll feel more confident in an emergency. When caring for a patient with a pacemaker, follow these guidelines.

For permanent pacemakers

◆ Use a systematic approach to assess pacemaker function for problems.
– What's the mode?
– What's the base rate and upper rate limit (maximum tracking or sensor rate)?
– Are such features as mode switching or rate response activated?
– Is the device a biventricular pacemaker?
– Is the patient pacemaker-dependent?
– Does the patient have signs and symptoms?

Oversensing
◆ Mistakes muscle movements or other events in cardiac cycle as intrinsic electrical activity
◆ Pacing won't occur when needed; heart rate and AV synchrony not maintained

Permanent pacemaker interventions
◆ Determine mode, base rate, and upper rate limit and if mode switching or rate response is activated

Permanent pacemaker interventions
(continued)

+ Evaluate all sources of information
+ Review patient's 12-lead ECG to evaluate pacemaker function
+ Select monitoring lead that shows pacemaker spikes, comparing at least two leads for verification
+ Measure rate; interpret paced rhythm
+ Compare morphology of paced and intrinsic complexes
+ Differentiate between ventricular ectopy and paced activity
+ Determine which chamber is paced and pacemaker's sensing function
+ Monitor patient's vital signs
+ Look for evidence of problems

Biventricular pacemaker interventions

+ Provide same basic care as that for standard permanent pacemaker
+ Because of left ventricular lead position, watch for stimulation of diaphragm and left chest wall
+ Observe for pacemaker spikes
+ Measure QRS complex duration

◆ Evaluate all sources of information:
– patient identification card issued by the pacemaker manufacturer
– patient history
– patient or family knowledge of device function
– physician notes, printouts from programmer if available
– ECG observation.
◆ Review the patient's 12-lead ECG to evaluate pacemaker function. If unavailable, examine lead V_1 or MCL_1 instead.
◆ Select a monitoring lead that clearly shows the pacemaker spikes and compare at least two leads to verify what you observe.
◆ Remember: Visibility of spikes depends on pacing polarity and type of lead.
◆ Measure the rate and interpret the paced rhythm.
◆ Compare the morphology of paced and intrinsic complexes (traditional right ventricular pacing should produce a morphology similar to left bundle-branch block pattern).
◆ Differentiate between ventricular ectopy and paced activity.
◆ Look for information that tells you which chamber is paced and information about the pacemaker's sensing function.
◆ Monitor the patient's vital signs.
◆ Look for evidence of problems:
– decreased cardiac output (hypotension, chest pain, dyspnea, syncope)
– infection
– pneumothorax
– abnormal electrical stimulation occurring in synchrony with the pacemaker
– pectoral muscle twitching
– hiccups (stimulation of diaphragm)
– cardiac tamponade.
◆ Placing a magnet over the pulse generator makes the pacemaker temporarily revert to an asynchronous mode (safety mode) at a preset rate. (See *Assessing pacemaker function.*)

For biventricular pacemakers

Provide the same basic care to the patient with a biventricular pacemaker that you would give a patient with a standard permanent pacemaker. Specific care includes these guidelines:
◆ Because of the position of the left ventricular lead, watch for stimulation of the diaphragm and left chest wall. Notify the physician if this occurs because the left ventricular lead may need repositioning.
◆ Observe the ECG for pacemaker spikes. Although both ventricles are paced, only one pacemaker spike is seen.

Assessing pacemaker function

When you apply a magnet to a pacemaker, the device reverts to a predefined (asynchronous) response mode that allows you to assess various aspects of pacemaker function. Specifically, you can accomplish the following:
+ Determine which chambers are being paced.
+ Assess capture.
+ Provide emergency pacing if the device malfunctions.
+ Ensure pacing despite electromagnetic interference.
+ Assess battery life by checking the magnet rate — a predetermined rate that indicates the need for battery replacement.

Keep in mind, however, that you must know which implanted device the patient has before you consider using a magnet on it. The patient might have an implantable cardioverter-defibrillator (ICD), which only rarely is an appropriate target for magnet application.

It used to be relatively easy to tell a pacemaker from an ICD because of the difference in generator size and implant location. Today it isn't as easy. The generators are similar in size, and both kinds of devices are implanted under the skin of the patient's chest. What's more, a single device may perform multiple functions.

In general, you shouldn't apply a magnet to an ICD or a pacemaker-ICD combination. Applying a magnet to an ICD can cause an unexpected response because various responses can be programmed or determined by the manufacturer. When directed, applying a magnet to an ICD usually suspends therapies for ventricular tachycardia and fibrillation while leaving bradycardia pacing active, which may be helpful in patients who receive multiple, inappropriate shocks. Some models may beep when exposed to a magnetic field.

+ Measure the duration of the QRS complex. Typically, you'll observe a narrowing of the QRS complex. A widened QRS complex may indicate that the left ventricular lead is no longer positioned properly.

For temporary pacemakers
+ Check stimulation and sensing thresholds daily because they increase over time.
+ Assess the patient and pacemaker regularly to check for possible problems:
– failure to capture
– undersensing
– oversensing.
+ Turn or reposition the patient carefully to prevent dislodgment of the leadwire.
+ Follow recommended electrical safety precautions.
+ Avoid microshocks to the patient by making sure that the bed and all electrical equipment is grounded properly and that all pacing wires and connections to temporary wires are insulated with moisture-proof material (such as a disposable glove).

Temporary pacemaker interventions
+ Check stimulation and sensing thresholds daily
+ Assess patient and pacemaker regularly
+ Turn or reposition patient to prevent dislodgement of leadwire
+ Follow recommended electrical safety precautions
+ Avoid microshocks by ensuring that all equipment is grounded and that all pacing wires and connections are insulated with moisture-proof material

Temporary pacemaker interventions
(continued)

+ Obtain chest X-ray and assist physician with repositioning of leadwire, if required
+ Invasive temporary pacing may deliver shock to heart along pacing wire, causing ventricular tachycardia or fibrillation
+ Defibrillation and cardioversion (up to 360 joules) don't usually require disconnection of pulse generator
+ Look for evidence of problems

+ Obtain a chest X-ray and assist the physician with repositioning the lead-wire if required.

Remember: All invasive temporary pacing has the potential to deliver a shock directly to the heart along the pacing wire, resulting in ventricular tachycardia or fibrillation.

+ Defibrillation and cardioversion (up to 360 joules) don't usually require that the pulse generator be disconnected.

+ Look for evidence of problems:
– decreased cardiac output (hypotension, chest pain, dyspnea, syncope)
– infection
– pneumothorax
– abnormal electrical stimulation occurring in synchrony with the pacemaker
– pectoral muscle twitching
– hiccups (stimulation of diaphragm)
– watch for signs of a perforated ventricle and the resultant cardiac tamponade. Signs and symptoms include persistent hiccups, tachycardia, distant heart sounds, pulsus paradoxus (a drop in the strength of a pulse during inspiration), hypotension with narrowed pulse pressure, cyanosis, distended jugular veins, decreased urine output, restlessness, and complaints of fullness in the chest. Notify the physician immediately if you note any of these signs and symptoms.

+ If there's no output (pacing is required but the pacemaker fails to stimulate the heart), take these steps:
– Verify that the pacemaker is on.
– Check the output settings.
– Change the pulse generator battery.
– Change the pulse generator.
– Check for disconnection or dislodgment of the pacing wire.

PATIENT EDUCATION

Following pacemaker insertion, explain why a pacemaker is needed, how it works, and what can be expected from it, be sure to cover these points with the patient and his family.

Permanent pacemaker teaching

+ Describe function, related anatomy and physiology, why it's needed, and postoperative care
+ Provide discharge instructions

For permanent pacemakers

+ Provide information to the patient about:
– pacemaker's function
– related anatomy and physiology
– patient's indication for pacemaker
– postoperative care and routines.
+ Provide discharge instructions, which usually include these topics:
– incision care

– signs of pocket complications (hematoma, infection, bleeding)
– avoidance of heavy lifting or vigorous activity for 2 to 4 weeks
– limited arm movement on side of pacemaker
– medical follow-up
– transtelephonic monitoring follow-up if indicated
– identification card to be carried
– procedure for taking pulse.

✦ Explain symptoms to report to physician:
– light-headedness, syncope, fatigue, palpitations, muscle stimulation, hiccups
– slow (below the base rate) or unusually fast heart rate.

✦ Because today's pacemakers are well shielded from environmental interactions, explain that the patient can safely use:
– most common household appliances, including microwaves
– cellular phones (on the opposite side of the device)
– spark-ignited combustion engines (leaf blower, lawnmower, automobile)
– office equipment (computer, copier, fax machine)
– light shop equipment.

✦ Caution the patient to avoid close or prolonged exposure to potential sources of electromagnetic interference. (See *Understanding EMI.*)

✦ Remind patient about travel-related issues:
– Metal detectors don't disturb device function but may detect the device.

Understanding EMI

Electromagnetic interference (EMI) can wreak havoc on patients who have a pacemaker or an implantable cardioverter-defibrillator (ICD). For someone with a pacemaker, EMI may inhibit pacing, cause asynchronous or unnecessary pacing, or mimic intrinsic cardiac activity. For someone with an ICD, EMI may mimic ventricular fibrillation, or it may prevent detection of a problem that needs treatment.

If your patient has a pacemaker or an ICD, review common sources of EMI and urge the patient to avoid them. These may include:
✦ strong electromagnetic fields
✦ large generators and transformers
✦ arc and resistance welders
✦ large magnets
✦ motorized radiofrequency equipment.

EMI may present a risk in medical or hospital settings as well. Make sure your patient knows to notify all health care providers about the implanted device so the provider can evaluate the risk of such therapies as:
✦ magnetic resonance imaging (usually contraindicated)
✦ radiation therapy (excluding diagnostic X-rays, such as mammograms, which typically are safe)
✦ diathermy
✦ electrocautery
✦ transcutaneous electrical nerve stimulation.

Permanent pacemaker teaching
(continued)

✦ Explain symptoms to report
✦ Explain that patient can use microwaves, cellular phones (on opposite side of device), and office and light shop equipment
✦ Caution patient to avoid exposure to potential sources of electromagnetic interference
✦ Remind patient that metal detectors won't disturb device; handheld scanners shouldn't be used near device

Understanding EMI

EMI sources to avoid
✦ Strong electromagnetic fields
✦ Large generators or transformers
✦ Arc and resistance welders
✦ Large magnets
✦ Motorized radiofrequency equipment

Therapies that may pose risk
✦ MRI
✦ Radiation therapy
✦ Diathermy
✦ Electrocautery
✦ TENS

– Handheld scanning tools shouldn't be used over the device or near it.
– An identification card may be needed to show security personnel.

Biventricular pacemaker teaching

- ◆ Provide same basic teaching as that for permanent pacemaker
- ◆ Explain function, why it's needed, and what to expect
- ◆ Explain symptoms to report

For biventricular pacemakers

Provide the same basic teaching that you would give to the patient receiving a permanent pacemaker. Additionally, when a patient gets a biventricular pacemaker, be sure to cover these points:

◆ Explain to the patient and his family why a biventricular pacemaker is needed, how it works, and what they can expect.

◆ Tell the patient and his family that it's sometimes difficult to place the left ventricular lead and that the procedure can take 3 hours or more.

◆ Stress the importance of calling the physician immediately if the patient develops chest pain, shortness of breath, swelling of the hands or feet, or a weight gain of 3 lb (1.4 kg) in 24 hours or 5 lb (2.3 kg) in 48 to 72 hours.

Temporary pacemaker teaching

- ◆ Explain function, related anatomy and physiology, and why it's needed
- ◆ Explain postprocedure care and pain management
- ◆ Advise patient not to get out of bed without assistance
- ◆ Explain symptoms to report
- ◆ Advise patient to limit arm movement on pacemaker side

For temporary pacemakers

◆ Provide information to the patient about the pacemaker's function, related anatomy and physiology, the need for the pacemaker, and potential need for a permanent pacemaker.

◆ Explain postprocedure care and pain management.

◆ Advise the patient not to get out of bed without assistance.

◆ Instruct the patient not to manipulate the pacemaker wires or pulse generator.

◆ Explain symptoms to report to the nurse: light-headedness, syncope, palpitations, muscle stimulation, or hiccups.

◆ Advise the patient to limit arm movement on the side of the pacemaker.

ICD

- ◆ Continuous monitoring for bradycardia and ventricular tachycardia and fibrillation
- ◆ Administers shocks or paced beats to treat dangerous arrhythmia
- ◆ Indicated when drug therapy, surgery, or catheter ablation has failed
- ◆ Insertion procedure similar to permanent pacemaker; may take place in cardiac catheterization lab

IMPLANTABLE CARDIOVERTER-DEFIBRILLATOR

An implantable cardioverter-defibrillator (ICD) is an electronic device implanted in the body to provide continuous monitoring of the heart for bradycardia, ventricular tachycardia, and ventricular fibrillation. The device then administers either shocks or paced beats to treat the dangerous arrhythmia. In general, ICDs are indicated for patients for whom drug therapy, surgery, or catheter ablation has failed to prevent the arrhythmia.

The procedure for ICD insertion is similar to that of a permanent pacemaker and may take place in a cardiac catheterization laboratory. Occasionally, a patient who requires other surgery, such as coronary artery bypass grafting, may have the device implanted in the operating room. (See *ICD review*.)

ICD review

Today's implantable cardioverter-defibrillators (ICDs) are easier to implant and more effective than ever. For most patients, the leads can be threaded through the cephalic vein and positioned in the heart and superior vena cava. The pulse generator is inserted under the skin through a small incision. In some cases, a high-voltage subcutaneous patch electrode is placed inside the superior periaxial area to reduce the amount of energy needed for defibrillation.

Programming features have evolved greatly and now allow tiered therapy, antitachycardia pacing, low-energy cardioversion, antibradycardia pacing, data storage, and diagnostic algorithms. In addition, some devices allow the magnet mode (in which placing a magnet over the generator suppresses ICD programming) to be turned on or off. With the magnet mode turned off, a magnet won't affect ICD function. In some devices, a magnet temporarily suspends detection and tachycardia therapy, while leaving antibradycardia pacing intact.

Originally, the only patients chosen to receive ICDs were those who survived sudden cardiac death and those who sustained ventricular tachycardia and syncope unresponsive to antiarrhythmic drugs. However, recent reports have revealed a survival rate 40% to 60% higher among at-risk patients with ICDs than among those who received conventional therapies. Consequently, ICDs are now recommended or being investigated for:
+ ventricular fibrillation without structural heart disease or triggering factors
+ syncope of an undetermined cause
+ unsuccessful antiarrhythmic therapy
+ patients with risk factors for ventricular arrhythmias
+ patients with extensive anterior wall myocardial infarction (MI) who can't take thrombolytic agents
+ patients with previous MI and unexplained recurrent syncope
+ children with congenital long QT-interval syndrome
+ patients who are waiting for heart transplantations.

An ICD consists of a programmable pulse generator and one or more leadwires. The pulse generator is a small battery-powered computer that monitors the heart's electrical signals and delivers electrical therapy when it identifies an abnormal rhythm. The leads are insulated wires that carry the heart signal to the pulse generator and deliver the electrical energy from the pulse generator to the heart.

An ICD also stores information about the heart's activity before, during, and after an arrhythmia, along with tracking which treatment was delivered and the treatment's outcome. Many devices also store electrograms (electrical tracings similar to ECGs). With an interrogation device, a physician can retrieve this information to evaluate ICD function and battery status and to adjust ICD system settings.

Today's advanced devices can detect a wide range of arrhythmias and automatically respond with the appropriate therapy, such as bradycardia pacing (both single- and dual-chamber), antitachycardia pacing, cardioversion, and defibrillation. ICDs that provide therapy for atrial arrhythmias, such as atrial fibrillation, are also available. (See *Types of ICD therapies,* page 190.)

ICD
(continued)
+ Consists of programmable pulse generator and one or more leadwires
+ Delivers electrical therapy for abnormal rhythms
+ Stores data about heart's electrical activity before, during, and after an arrhythmia; also tracks treatment and outcome
+ Data can be retrieved to evaluate ICD function and battery status and adjust system settings

Types of ICD therapies

An implantable cardioverter-defibrillator (ICD) can deliver a range of therapies depending on the type of device, how the device is programmed and the arrhythmia it detects. Therapies include antitachycardia pacing, cardioversion, defibrillation, and bradycardia pacing.

THERAPY	DESCRIPTION
Antitachycardia pacing	A series of small, rapid electrical pacing pulses used to interrupt atrial fibrillation (AF) or ventricular tachycardia (VT) and return the heart to its normal rhythm. Antitachycardia pacing isn't appropriate for all patients and begins only after appropriate electrophysiology studies.
Cardioversion	A low- or high-energy shock (up to 35 joules) timed to the R wave to terminate VT and return the heart to its normal rhythm.
Defibrillation	A high-energy shock (up to 35 joules) to the heart to terminate ventricular fibrillation or AF and return the heart to its normal rhythm.
Bradycardia pacing	Electrical pacing pulses used when natural electrical signals are too slow. Most ICDs pace one chamber (VVI pacing) of the heart at a preset rate. Some can sense and pace both chambers (DDD pacing).

Interventions

+ Know how device is programmed including type and model, device status, detection rates, and therapies to be delivered
+ If arrhythmia occurs, assess patient, record ECG rhythm, and evaluate ICD response
+ Initiate CPR or ACLS if patient experiences cardiac arrest
+ Don't place paddles directly over pulse generator when externally defibrillating patient

INTERVENTIONS

When caring for a patient with an ICD, it's important to know how the device is programmed. This information is available through a status report that can be obtained and printed when the physician or specially trained technician interrogates the device. This involves placing a specialized piece of equipment over the implanted pulse generator to retrieve pacing function. If the patient experiences an arrhythmia or the ICD delivers a therapy, the program information recorded helps to evaluate the functioning of the device.

Program information includes:
+ type and model of ICD
+ status of the device (on or off)
+ detection rates
+ therapies that will be delivered: pacing, antitachycardia pacing, cardioversion, and defibrillation.

If your patient experiences an arrhythmia:
+ Assess the patient for signs and symptoms related to decreased cardiac output.
+ Record the patient's ECG rhythm.
+ Evaluate the appropriateness of any delivered ICD therapy.
+ If the patient experiences cardiac arrest, initiate cardiopulmonary resuscitation (CPR) and advanced cardiac life support (ACLS).

✦ If the patient needs external defibrillation, position the paddles as far from the device as possible or use the anteroposterior paddle position.

PATIENT EDUCATION

✦ Explain to the patient and his family why an ICD is needed, how it works, potential complications, and what they can expect. Make sure they also understand ICD terminology.

✦ Discuss signs and symptoms to report to the physician immediately.

✦ Advise the patient to wear a medical identification bracelet indicating ICD placement.

✦ Educate family members in emergency techniques (such as dialing 911 and performing CPR) in case the device fails.

✦ Explain that electrical or electronic devices may cause disruption of the device.

✦ Warn the patient to avoid placing excessive pressure over the insertion site or moving or jerking the area until the postoperative visit.

✦ Tell the patient to follow normal routines as allowed by the physician and to increase exercise as tolerated. After the first 24 hours, show the patient how to perform passive range-of-motion exercises and progress as tolerated.

✦ Remind the patient to carry information regarding his ICD at all times and to inform airline clerks when he travels as well as individuals performing diagnostic functions (such as computed tomography scans and magnetic resonance imaging).

✦ Stress the importance of follow-up care and checkups.

RADIOFREQUENCY ABLATION

Radiofrequency ablation is an invasive procedure that may be used to treat arrhythmias in patients who haven't responded to antiarrhythmic drugs or cardioversion or can't tolerate antiarrhythmic drugs. In this procedure, a burst of radiofrequency energy is delivered through a catheter to the heart tissue to destroy the arrhythmia's focus or block the conduction pathway.

Radiofrequency ablation is effective in treating patients with atrial fibrillation and flutter, ventricular tachycardia, AV nodal reentry tachycardia, and Wolff-Parkinson-White (WPW) syndrome.

PROCEDURE

The patient first undergoes electrophysiology studies to identify and map the specific area of the heart that's causing the arrhythmia. The ablation catheters are inserted into a vein, usually the femoral vein, and advanced to the heart where short bursts of radiofrequency waves destroy a small targeted

Patient education

✦ Explain to patient and family why ICD is needed, how it works, and what to expect
✦ Discuss signs and symptoms to report immediately
✦ Advise patient to wear medical ID bracelet
✦ Educate family in emergency techniques
✦ Warn patient to avoid placing excessive pressure over insertion site
✦ Tell patient to follow normal routines as allowed by physician
✦ Remind patient to always carry information regarding ICD
✦ Stress importance of follow-up care

Radiofrequency ablation

✦ Treats arrhythmias in patients who haven't responded to antiarrhythmic drugs
✦ Energy delivered to destroy arrhythmia or block conduction pathway

Procedure

✦ Electrophysiology first to identify area that's causing arrhythmia
✦ Catheter inserted into vein (usually femoral) and advanced to heart

Procedure
(continued)

◆ Radiofrequency waves destroy targeted area of tissue, preventing it from conducting impulses

◆ If arrhythmia develops above AV node, AV nodal ablation may be used

◆ Permanent pacemaker may then be needed as impulses can't be conducted from atria to ventricles

Interventions

◆ Monitor for arrhythmias and ischemic changes

◆ Place on bed rest for 8 hours, keeping affected extremity straight

◆ Maintain head of bed between 15 and 30 degrees

◆ Check vital signs every 15 minutes for first hour, then every 30 minutes for 4 hours

◆ Assess peripheral pulses distal to insertion site

◆ Monitor site for bleeding and hematoma and patient for complications

Patient education

◆ Discuss why radiofrequency ablation is needed, how it works, and what to expect

◆ Warn that procedure can take up to 6 hours and that hospitalization ranges from 24 to 48 hours

area of heart tissue. The destroyed tissue can no longer conduct electrical impulses. Other types of energy may also be used, such as microwave, sonar, or cryo (freezing). In some patients, the tissue inside the pulmonary vein is responsible for the arrhythmia. Targeted radiofrequency ablation is used to block these abnormal impulses. (See *Destroying the source.*)

If a rapid arrhythmia that originates above the AV node (such as atrial fibrillation) isn't terminated by targeted ablation, AV nodal ablation may be used to block electrical impulses from being conducted to the ventricles. After ablation of the AV node, the patient may need a pacemaker because impulses can no longer be conducted from the atria to the ventricles. If the atria continue to beat irregularly, anticoagulation therapy will also be needed to reduce the risk of stroke.

If the patient has WPW syndrome, electrophysiology studies can locate the accessory pathway and ablation can destroy it. When reentry is the cause of the arrhythmia, such as AV nodal reentry tachycardia, ablation can destroy the pathway without affecting the AV node.

INTERVENTIONS

When caring for a patient after radiofrequency ablation, follow these guidelines:

◆ Provide continuous cardiac monitoring, assessing for arrhythmias and ischemic changes.

◆ Place the patient on bed rest for 8 hours, or as ordered, and keep the affected extremity straight. Maintain the head of the bed between 15 and 30 degrees.

◆ Assess the patient's vital signs every 15 minutes for the first hour, then every 30 minutes for 4 hours, unless the patient's condition warrants more frequent checking.

◆ Assess peripheral pulses distal to the catheter insertion site as well as the color, sensation, temperature, and capillary refill of the affected extremity.

◆ Check the catheter insertion site for bleeding and hematoma formation.

◆ Monitor the patient for complications, such as hemorrhage, stroke, perforation of the heart, arrhythmias, phrenic nerve damage, pericarditis, pulmonary vein stenosis or thrombosis, and sudden death.

PATIENT EDUCATION

When a patient undergoes radiofrequency ablation, be sure to cover these points:

◆ Discuss with the patient and his family why radiofrequency ablation is needed, how it works, and what they can expect.

◆ Warn the patient and his family that the procedure can be lengthy, up to 6 hours if electrophysiology studies are being done first.

Destroying the source

In radiofrequency ablation, special catheters are inserted in a vein and advanced to the heart. After the arrhythmia's source is identified, radiofrequency energy is used to destroy the source of the abnormal electrical impulses or abnormal conduction pathway.

AV NODAL ABLATION

If a rapid arrhythmia originates above the atrioventricular (AV) node, the AV node may be destroyed to block impulses from reaching the ventricles. The radiofrequency ablation catheter is directed to the AV node (A). Radiofrequency energy is used to destroy the AV node (B).

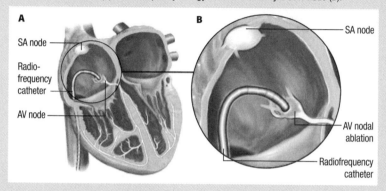

PULMONARY VEIN ABLATION

If the pulmonary vein is the source of the arrhythmia, radiofrequency energy is used to destroy the tissue at the base of the pulmonary vein. The radiofrequency catheter is directed to the base of the pulmonary vein (A). Radiofrequency energy is used to destroy the tissue at the base of the pulmonary vein (B).

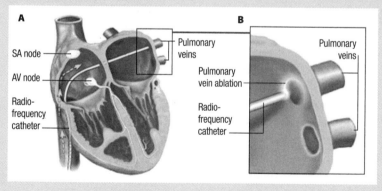

♦ Explain that the patient may be hospitalized for 24 to 48 hours to monitor his heart rhythm.

♦ Provide pacemaker teaching if the patient had a pacemaker inserted.

VENTRICULAR ASSIST DEVICES

Ventricular assist devices

- ♦ Decrease heart's workload and increase cardiac output
- ♦ Right VAD diverts blood from right ventricle to VAD, which pumps it back to body via pulmonary artery
- ♦ Left VAD diverts blood from left ventricle to VAD, which pumps it back to body via aorta

Ventricular assist devices (VADs) are designed to decrease the heart's workload and increase cardiac output in patients with ventricular failure. Left ventricular, right ventricular, and biventricular VADs are available. (See *VAD: Help for a failing heart.*)

Because a VAD supports the heart's pumping function rather than altering electrical function, it doesn't affect the heart's electrical activity. As a result, you probably won't see ECG changes caused by the VAD.

VADs may be indicated for patients who can't be weaned from cardiopulmonary bypass or intra-aortic balloon pump as well as for patients who are awaiting heart transplantation.

In a surgical procedure, blood is diverted from a ventricle to an artificial pump, which maintains systemic perfusion. VADs are commonly used as a bridge to maintain perfusion until a heart transplantation procedure can be performed.

A VAD is used to provide systemic or pulmonary support, or both:

♦ A right VAD provides pulmonary support by diverting blood from the failing right ventricle to the VAD, which then pumps the blood to the pulmonary circulation by way of the VAD connection to the pulmonary artery.

♦ With a left VAD, blood flows from the left ventricle to the VAD, which then pumps blood back to the body by way of the VAD connection to the aorta.

♦ When biventricular support is needed, both may be used.

INTERVENTIONS

Interventions

Patient preparation
- ♦ Prepare patient and family for insertion
- ♦ Ensure that informed consent is obtained
- ♦ Continue close patient monitoring

Monitoring and aftercare
- ♦ Assess cardiovascular status
- ♦ Inspect incision and dressing

Patient preparation

♦ Prepare the patient and his family for insertion, reinforcing explanations about the device, its purpose, and what to expect after insertion.

♦ Make sure that informed consent is obtained.

♦ Continue close patient monitoring, including continuous ECG monitoring, pulmonary artery and hemodynamic status monitoring, and intake and output monitoring.

Monitoring and aftercare

♦ Assess the patient's cardiovascular status, monitor blood pressure and hemodynamic parameters, including cardiac output and cardiac index, ECG, and peripheral pulses.

VAD: Help for a failing heart

A ventricular assist device (VAD), which is commonly called a *bridge to transplant,* is a mechanical pump that relieves the ventricle's workload as the heart heals or until a donor heart is located.

IMPLANTABLE

The typical VAD is implanted in the upper abdominal wall. An inflow cannula drains blood from the left ventricle into a pump, which then pushes the blood into the aorta through the outflow cannula.

PUMP OPTIONS

VADs are available as continuous-flow or pulsatile pumps. A *continuous-flow pump* fills continuously and returns blood to the aorta at a constant rate. A *pulsatile pump* may work in one of two ways: It may fill during systole and pump blood into the aorta during diastole, or it may pump irrespective of the patient's cardiac cycle.

Many types of VAD systems are available. This illustration shows a VAD (from Baxter Novacor) implanted in the left abdominal wall and connected to an external controller by a percutaneous lead. The patient also has a reserve power pack. The monitor is a backup power source that can run on electricity.

POTENTIAL COMPLICATIONS

Despite the use of anticoagulants, the VAD may cause thrombi formation, leading to pulmonary embolism or stroke. Other complications may include heart failure, bleeding, cardiac tamponade, or infection.

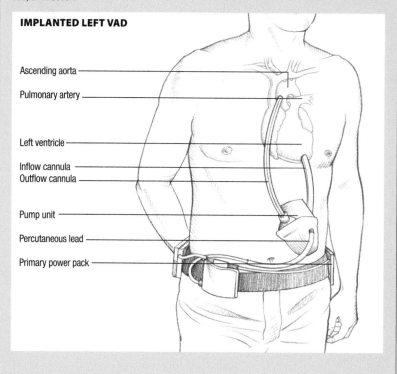

IMPLANTED LEFT VAD

Ascending aorta

Pulmonary artery

Left ventricle

Inflow cannula
Outflow cannula

Pump unit

Percutaneous lead

Primary power pack

Interventions
(continued)

Monitoring and aftercare
+ Monitor urine output hourly; maintain I.V. fluid therapy
+ Assess chest tube drainage and function
+ Evaluate oxygen saturation or mixed venous oxygen saturation levels
+ Obtain Hb levels, HCT, and coagulation studies
+ Administer blood and antibiotics, as ordered

Patient education

Instruct patient to:
+ report redness, swelling, or drainage at incision site; and chest pain or fever
+ report signs and symptoms of heart failure
+ follow prescribed medication and diet regimen
+ maintain balance between activity and rest
+ follow rehabilitation program
+ comply with lab schedule (if receiving warfarin)

+ Inspect the incision and dressing at least every hour initially and then every 2 to 4 hours as indicated by the patient's condition.
+ Monitor urine output hourly, and maintain I.V. fluid therapy as ordered. Watch for signs of fluid overload or decreasing urine output.
+ Assess chest tube drainage and function frequently. Notify the physician if drainage is greater than 150 ml over 2 hours. Auscultate lungs for evidence of abnormal breath sounds. Evaluate oxygen saturation or mixed venous oxygen saturation levels, and administer oxygen as needed and ordered.
+ Obtain hemoglobin (Hb) levels, hematocrit (HCT), and coagulation studies as ordered. Administer blood component therapy as indicated and ordered.
+ Assess for signs and symptoms of bleeding.
+ Administer antibiotics prophylactically if ordered.

PATIENT EDUCATION

Before discharge after the insertion of a VAD, instruct the patient to:
+ immediately report redness, swelling, or drainage at the incision site; chest pain; or fever
+ immediately notify the physician if signs or symptoms of heart failure (weight gain, dyspnea, or edema) develop
+ follow the prescribed medication regimen and report adverse effects
+ follow his prescribed diet, especially sodium and fat restrictions
+ maintain a balance between activity and rest
+ follow his exercise or rehabilitation program (if prescribed)
+ comply with the laboratory schedule for monitoring International Normalized Ratio if the patient is receiving warfarin (Coumadin).

Basic 12-lead ECG

The 12-lead electrocardiogram (ECG) is a diagnostic test that helps identify pathologic conditions, especially ischemia and acute myocardial infarction (MI). It provides a more complete view of the heart's electrical activity than a rhythm strip and can be used to assess left ventricular function more effectively. Patients with conditions that affect the heart's electrical system may also benefit from a 12-lead ECG, including those with:

+ cardiac arrhythmias
+ heart chamber enlargement or hypertrophy
+ digoxin or other drug toxicity
+ electrolyte imbalances
+ pulmonary embolism
+ pericarditis
+ pacemakers
+ hypothermia.

Like other diagnostic tests, a 12-lead ECG must be viewed in conjunction with other clinical data. Therefore, always correlate the patient's ECG results with the history, physical assessment findings, and results of laboratory and other diagnostic studies as well as the drug regimen.

Remember, too, that an ECG can be done in various ways, including over a telephone line. (See *Transtelephonic cardiac monitoring,* page 198.) In fact, transtelephonic monitoring has become increasingly important as a tool for assessing patients at home and in other nonclinical settings.

The 12-lead ECG records the heart's electrical activity using a series of electrodes placed on the patient's extremities and chest wall. The 12 leads in-

Basic 12-lead ECG
+ Helps identify pathologic conditions (ischemia, acute MI)
+ Provides better view of electrical activity than rhythm strip
+ Assesses left ventricular function more effectively
+ Results examined in conjunction with other clinical data

Leads
+ Three bipolar limb (I, II, III)
+ Three unipolar augmented limb (aV_R, aV_L, aV_F)
+ Six unipolar precordial or chest (V_1 to V_6)

TTM

+ Allows patients to transmit ECGs (when symptoms appear) by phone
+ Enables health care professional to assess transient conditions that cause symptoms

Home care

+ Appropriate also for patient undergoing cardiac rehab
+ Valuable for assessing effects of drugs and diagnosing and managing paroxysmal arrhythmias

Understanding TTM equipment

+ Three main pieces: ECG recorder-transmitter, standard phone line, and receiver

Credit card-size recorder

+ Battery operated; stores 30 seconds of activity, later transmitting across phone lines

---

Transtelephonic cardiac monitoring

Using a special recorder-transmitter, patients at home can transmit ECGs by telephone to a central monitoring center for immediate interpretation. This technique, called *transtelephonic cardiac monitoring* (TTM), reduces health care costs and is being used more often.

Nurses play an important role in TTM. Besides performing extensive patient and family teaching, they may operate the central monitoring center and help interpret ECGs sent by patients.

TTM allows a health care professional to assess transient conditions that cause such symptoms as palpitations, dizziness, syncope, confusion, paroxysmal dyspnea, and chest pain. Such conditions, which are commonly not apparent while the patient is with a health care professional, can make diagnosis difficult and costly.

With TTM, the patient can transmit an ECG recording from his home when the symptoms appear, avoiding the need to go to the hospital and offering a greater opportunity for early diagnosis. Even if symptoms seldom appear, the patient can keep the equipment for long periods, which further aids in the diagnosis of the patient's condition.

HOME CARE

TTM can also be used by a patient having cardiac rehabilitation at home. He'll be called regularly during this period to assess his progress. Because of this continuous monitoring, TTM can help reduce the anxiety felt by the patient and his family after discharge, especially if the patient suffered a myocardial infarction.

TTM is especially valuable for assessing the effects of drugs and for diagnosing and managing paroxysmal arrhythmias. In both cases, TTM can eliminate the need for admitting the patient for evaluation and a potentially lengthy hospital stay.

UNDERSTANDING TTM EQUIPMENT

TTM requires three main pieces of equipment: an ECG recorder-transmitter, a standard telephone line, and a receiver. The ECG recorder-transmitter converts electrical activity from the patient's heart into acoustic waves. Some models contain built-in memory devices that store recordings of cardiac activity for transmission later.

A standard telephone line is used to transmit information. The receiver converts the acoustic waves transmitted over the telephone line into ECG activity, which is then recorded on ECG paper for interpretation and documentation in the patient's chart. The recorder-transmitter uses two types of electrodes applied to the finger and chest. The electrodes produce ECG tracings similar to those of a standard 12-lead ECG.

CREDIT CARD-SIZE RECORDER

One recently developed recorder operates on a battery and is about the size of a credit card. When a patient becomes symptomatic, he holds the back of the card firmly to the center of his chest and pushes the start button. Four electrodes located on the back of the card sense electrical activity and record it. The card can store 30 seconds of activity and can later transmit the recording across phone lines for evaluation by a clinician.

---

clude three bipolar limb leads (I, II, III), three unipolar augmented limb leads (aV_R, aV_L, and aV_F), and six unipolar precordial, or chest, leads (V_1, V_2, V_3, V_4, V_5, and V_6). These leads provide 12 different views of the heart's electrical activity. (See *ECG leads.*)

Scanning up, down, and across, each lead transmits information about a different area of the heart. The waveforms obtained from each lead vary de-

ECG leads

Each of the leads on a 12-lead ECG views the heart from a different angle. These illustrations show the direction of electrical activity (depolarization) monitored by each lead and the 12 views of the heart.

VIEWS REFLECTED ON A 12-LEAD ECG	LEAD	VIEW OF THE HEART
	Standard limb leads (bipolar)	
	I	lateral wall
	II	inferior wall
	III	inferior wall
	Augmented limb leads (unipolar)	
	aV_R	no specific view
	aV_L	lateral wall
	aV_F	inferior wall
	Precordial, or chest, leads (unipolar)	
	V_1	septal wall
	V_2	septal wall
	V_3	anterior wall
	V_4	anterior wall
	V_5	lateral wall
	V_6	lateral wall

pending on the lead's location in relation to the wave of depolarization passing through the myocardium.

LIMB LEADS

The six limb leads record electrical activity in the heart's frontal plane, a view through the middle of the heart from top to bottom. Electrical activity is recorded from the anterior to the posterior axes.

Limb leads
+ Record electrical activity in heart's frontal plane

Precordial leads
+ Provide data on electrical activity in heart's horizontal plane

PRECORDIAL LEADS

The six precordial leads provide information on electrical activity in the heart's horizontal plane, a transverse view through the middle of the heart, dividing it into upper and lower portions. Electrical activity is recorded from either a superior or an inferior approach.

Electrical axes
+ In healthy heart, impulses move downward and to left (direction of normal axis)
+ In unhealthy heart, impulses travel away from damage or necrosis and toward areas of hypertrophy (axis direction varied)

ELECTRICAL AXES

As well as assessing 12 different leads, a 12-lead ECG records the heart's electrical axis. The term axis refers to the direction of depolarization as it spreads through the heart. As impulses travel through the heart, they generate small electrical forces called instantaneous vectors. The mean of these vectors represents the force and direction of the wave of depolarization through the heart—the electrical axis. The electrical axis is also called the mean instantaneous vector and the mean QRS vector.

In a healthy heart, impulses originate in the sinoatrial node, travel through the atria to the atrioventricular node, and then to the ventricles. Most of the movement of the impulses is downward and to the left, the direction of a normal axis.

In an unhealthy heart, axis direction varies. That's because the direction of electrical activity travels away from areas of damage or necrosis and toward areas of hypertrophy. Knowing the normal deflection of each lead will help you evaluate whether the electrical axis is normal or abnormal.

OBTAINING A 12-LEAD ECG

To perform a 12-lead ECG, you'll need to prepare properly, select the appropriate electrode sites, understand how to perform variations on a standard 12-lead ECG, and make an accurate recording.

Preparation
+ Gather ECG machine, recording paper, electrodes, and gauze pads
+ Inform patient that ECG has been ordered and explain procedure
+ Ask patient to lie in supine position; if he can't lie flat, raise bed to semi-Fowler's position
+ Document position during procedure

PREPARATION

Gather all necessary supplies, including the ECG machine, recording paper, electrodes, and gauze pads. Tell the patient that the physician has ordered an ECG, and explain the procedure. Emphasize that the test takes about 10 minutes and that it's a safe and painless way to evaluate the heart's electrical activity. Answer the patient's questions, and offer reassurance. Preparing the patient properly will help alleviate anxiety and promote cooperation.

Ask the patient to lie in a supine position in the center of the bed with arms at his sides. If he can't tolerate lying flat, raise the head of the bed to semi-Fowler's position. Document the patient's position during the procedure. Ensure privacy, and expose the patient's arms, legs, and chest, draping for comfort.

SITE SELECTION

Select the areas where you'll apply the electrodes. Choose areas that are flat and fleshy and not muscular or bony. Clip the area if it's excessively hairy. Remove excess oil and other substances from the skin to enhance electrode contact. Remember, the better the electrode contact, the better the recording.

The 12-lead ECG provides 12 different views of the heart, just as 12 photographers snapping the same picture would produce 12 different photographs. Taking all of those snapshots requires placing four electrodes on the limbs and six across the front of the chest wall.

To help ensure an accurate recording, the electrodes must be applied correctly. Inaccurate placement of an electrode by greater than $5/8''$ (1.5 cm) from its standardized position may lead to inaccurate waveforms and an incorrect ECG interpretation.

 AGE CHANGE You'll need patience when obtaining a pediatric ECG. With the help of the parents, if possible, try distracting the attention of a child. If artifact from arm and leg movement is a problem, try placing the electrodes in a more proximal position on the extremity.

Limb lead placement

To record the bipolar limb leads I, II, and III and the unipolar limb leads aV_R, aV_L, and aV_F, place electrodes on both of the patient's arms and on his left leg. The right leg also receives an electrode, but that electrode acts as a ground and doesn't contribute to the waveform. (See *Limb lead placement*, page 202.)

Placing the electrodes on the patient is typically easy because each lead-wire is labeled or color-coded. For example, a wire (usually white) might be labeled "RA" for right arm. Another (usually red) might be labeled "LL" for left leg.

Precordial lead placement

Precordial leads are also labeled or color coded according to which wire corresponds to which lead. To record the six precordial leads (V_1 through V_6), position the electrodes on specific areas of the anterior chest wall. (See *Precordial lead placement*, page 203.) If they're placed too low, the ECG tracing will be inaccurate.

✦ Place lead V_1 over the fourth intercostal space at the right sternal border. To find the space, locate the sternal notch at the second rib and feel your way down the sternal border until you reach the fourth intercostal space.

Site selection
✦ Select areas for electrodes, choosing flat and fleshy areas (if excessively hairy, clip)
✦ Remove excess oil for better recording
✦ Place electrodes accurately to prevent altered waveforms and incorrect interpretation

Limb lead placement
✦ For bipolar and unipolar limb leads, place electrodes on both arms and left leg
✦ Electrode on right leg acts as ground and doesn't affect waveform

Precordial lead placement
✦ For precordial leads, place electrodes on specific anterior chest wall areas

Limb lead placement

Proper lead placement is critical for the accurate recording of cardiac rhythms. The diagrams here show electrode placement for the six limb leads. RA indicates right arm; LA, left arm; RL, right leg; and LL, left leg. The plus sign (+) indicates the positive pole, the minus sign (–) indicates the negative pole, and G indicates the ground. Below each diagram is a sample ECG recording for that lead.

LEAD I
Lead I connects the right arm (negative pole) with the left arm (positive pole).

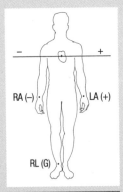

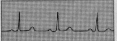

LEAD II
Lead II connects the right arm (negative pole) with the left leg (positive pole).

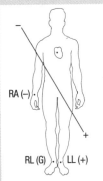

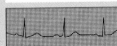

LEAD III
Lead III connects the left arm (negative pole) with the left leg (positive pole).

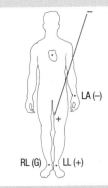

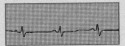

LEAD AV_R
Lead aV_R connects the right arm (positive pole) with the heart (negative pole).

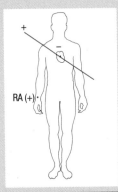

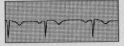

LEAD AV_L
Lead aV_L connects the left arm (positive pole) with the heart (negative pole).

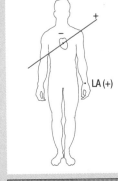

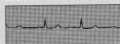

LEAD AV_F
Lead aV_F connects the left leg (positive pole) with the heart (negative pole).

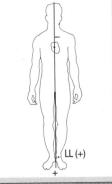

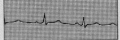

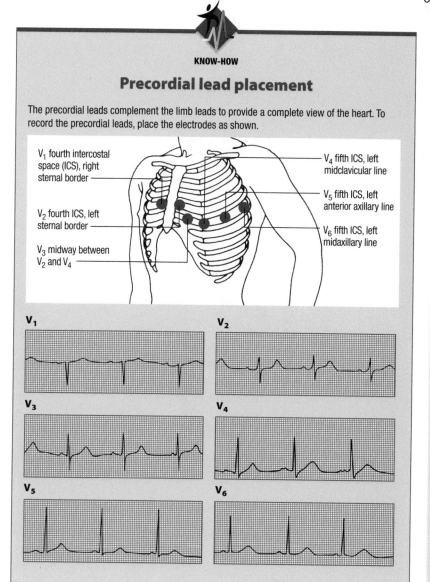

KNOW-HOW

Precordial lead placement

The precordial leads complement the limb leads to provide a complete view of the heart. To record the precordial leads, place the electrodes as shown.

V_1 fourth intercostal space (ICS), right sternal border

V_2 fourth ICS, left sternal border

V_3 midway between V_2 and V_4

V_4 fifth ICS, left midclavicular line

V_5 fifth ICS, left anterior axillary line

V_6 fifth ICS, left midaxillary line

V_1 V_2

V_3 V_4

V_5 V_6

✦ Place lead V_2 just opposite V_1, over the fourth intercostal space at the left sternal border.

✦ Place lead V_4 over the fifth intercostal space at the left midclavicular line. Placing lead V_4 before V_3 makes it easier to see where to place lead V_3.

✦ Place lead V_3 midway between V_2 and V_4.

✦ Place lead V_5 over the fifth intercostal space at the left anterior axillary line.

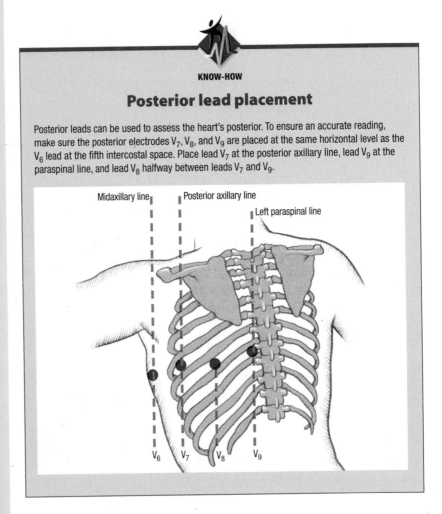

Posterior lead placement

Posterior leads can be used to assess the heart's posterior. To ensure an accurate reading, make sure the posterior electrodes V_7, V_8, and V_9 are placed at the same horizontal level as the V_6 lead at the fifth intercostal space. Place lead V_7 at the posterior axillary line, lead V_9 at the paraspinal line, and lead V_8 halfway between leads V_7 and V_9.

✦ Place lead V_6 over the fifth intercostal space at the left midaxillary line. If you've placed leads V_4 through V_6 correctly, they should line up horizontally.

Additional types of ECGs

In addition to the standard 12-lead ECG, two other types of ECGs may be used for diagnostic purposes: the posterior-lead ECG and the right chest lead ECG. These ECGs use chest leads to assess areas that standard 12-lead ECGs can't.

Posterior-lead ECG

Because of lung and muscle barriers, the usual chest leads can't "see" the heart's posterior surface to record myocardial damage there. So some physicians add three posterior leads to the 12-lead ECG: leads V_7, V_8, and V_9. These leads are placed opposite anterior leads V_4, V_5, and V_6, on the left side

Posterior-lead ECG

✦ Three posterior leads (V_7, V_8, V_9)
✦ Due to lung and muscle, may be added to heart's posterior surface to record damage

of the patient's back, following the same horizontal line. (See *Posterior lead placement*.)

Occasionally, a physician may request right-sided posterior leads. These leads are labeled V_{7R}, V_{8R}, and V_{9R} and are placed on the right side of the patient's back. Their placement is a mirror image of the electrodes on the left side of the back. This type of ECG provides information on the right posterior area of the heart.

Right chest lead ECG

The standard 12-lead ECG evaluates only the left ventricle. If the right ventricle needs to be assessed for damage or dysfunction, the physician may order a right chest lead ECG. For example, a patient with an inferior wall MI might have a right chest lead ECG to rule out right ventricular involvement.

With this type of ECG, the six leads are placed on the right side of the chest in a mirror image of the standard precordial lead placement. Electrodes start at the left sternal border and swing down under the right breast area (See *Right precordial lead placement*, page 206.)

RECORDING THE ECG

After properly placing the electrodes, record the ECG. ECG machines come in two types: multichannel recorders (most common) and single-channel recorders. With a multichannel recorder, all electrodes are attached to the patient at once and the machine prints a simultaneous view of all leads. With a single-channel recorder, one lead at a time is recorded in a short strip by attaching and removing electrodes and stopping and starting the tracing each time.

To record a multichannel ECG, follow these steps:

✦ Plug the cord of the ECG machine into a grounded outlet. If the machine operates on a charged battery, it may not need to be plugged in.

✦ Place all of the electrodes on the patient.

✦ Make sure all leads are securely attached, and then turn on the machine.

✦ Instruct the patient to relax, lie still, and breathe normally. Ask him not to talk during the recording, to prevent distortion of the ECG tracing.

✦ Set the ECG paper speed selector to 25 mm per second. If necessary, enter the patient's identification data.

✦ Press the appropriate button on the ECG machine and record the ECG.

✦ Observe the quality of the tracing. When the machine finishes the recording, turn it off.

✦ Remove the electrodes, and clean the patient's skin.

Right chest lead ECG

✦ Right chest lead may be ordered to assess right ventricle

✦ Six leads placed on right side of the chest in mirror image of standard precordial leads

✦ Electrodes start at left sternal border down to area under right breast

Recording the ECG

✦ *Multichannel recorder*—Prints simultaneous view of all leads

✦ *Single-channel recorder*—One lead at a time is recorded in short strip

Follow these steps:

✦ Plug cord into grounded outlet, if machine doesn't operate on charged battery

✦ Place electrodes on the patient, making sure that leads are secure, and turn on machine

✦ Ask patient not to talk during recording, to prevent distortion

✦ Set paper speed selector to 25 mm/second

✦ Enter patient's data

✦ Press appropriate button and record

✦ Observe quality of tracing

✦ Remove electrodes; clean patient's skin

Right precordial lead placement

Right precordial leads can provide specific information about the function of the right ventricle. Place the six leads on the right side of the chest in a mirror image of the standard precordial lead placement, as shown here.

V_1R: fourth intercostal space (ICS), left sternal border
V_2R: fourth ICS, right sternal border
V_3R: halfway between V_2R and V_4R
V_4R: fifth ICS, right midclavicular line
V_5R: fifth ICS, right anterior axillary line
V_6R: fifth ICS, right midaxillary line

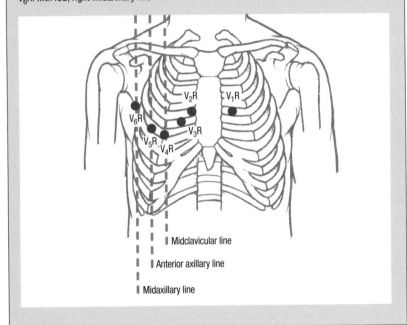

ECG recording

+ Tracing shows patient's name, room number, and medical record number (possibly)
+ Some machines can record ST-segment elevation and depression
+ Date, time, physician's name, and special circumstances must be written on printout

ECG RECORDING

Depending on the information entered, ECG printouts from a multichannel ECG machine will show the patient's name and room number and, possibly, his medical record number. At the top of the printout, you'll see the patient's heart rate and wave durations, measured in seconds. (See *Multichannel ECG recording.*)

Some machines can record ST-segment elevation and depression. The name of the lead will appear next to each 6-second strip.

Multichannel ECG recording

The top of a 12-lead ECG recording usually shows patient identification information along with an interpretation by the machine. A rhythm strip is commonly included at the bottom of the recording.

STANDARDIZATION

Look for standardization marks on the recording, normally 10 small squares high. If the patient has high voltage complexes, the marks will be half as high. You'll also notice that lead markers separate the lead recordings on the paper and that each lead is labeled.

Familiarize yourself with the order in which the leads are arranged on an ECG tracing. Getting accustomed to the layout of the tracing will help you interpret the ECG more quickly and accurately.

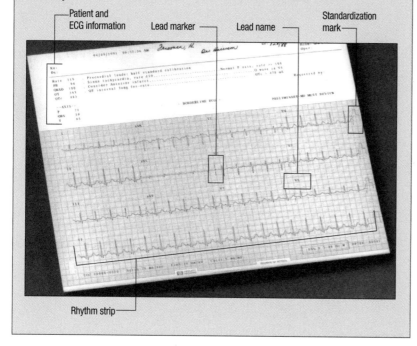

Patient and ECG information · Lead marker · Lead name · Standardization mark · Rhythm strip

If not already included on the printout, be sure to write the following information: date, time, physician's name, and special circumstances. For example, you might record an episode of chest pain, abnormal electrolyte levels, related drug treatment, abnormal placement of the electrodes, or the presence of an artificial pacemaker and whether a magnet was used while the ECG was obtained.

Remember, ECGs are legal documents. They belong in the patient's medical record and must be saved for future reference and comparison with baseline strips.

Advanced electrocardiography

With an electrocardiogram (ECG) in hand, the final skill involves interpreting the rhythm and understanding how various disorders can affect those interpretations. This chapter examines ECG interpretation and variations in such disorders as angina, bundle-branch block, myocardial infarction, pericarditis, Prinzmetal's angina, and left ventricular hypertrophy.

INTERPRETING ECGS

To interpret a 12-lead ECG, use a systematic approach. Compare the patient's previous ECG with the current one, if available. This will help you identify changes.

STEPS IN INTERPRETATION

1. Check the ECG tracing to see if it's technically correct. Make sure the baseline is free from electrical interference and drift.
2. Scan the limb leads I, II, and III. The R-wave voltage in lead II should equal the sum of the R-wave voltage in leads I and III. Lead aV$_R$ is typically negative. If these rules aren't met, the tracing may be recorded incorrectly.
3. Locate the lead markers on the waveform. Lead markers are the points where one lead changes to another.
4. Check the standardization markings (1 millivolt or 10 mm) to make sure all leads were recorded with the ECG machine's amplitude at the same set-

Interpreting ECGs
✦ Compare patient's previous ECG with current one

Steps in interpretation
✦ Check tracing for accuracy
✦ Scan limb leads, locating lead markers on waveform
✦ Check standardization markings (1 millivolt or 10 mm)

Steps in interpretation
(continued)

+ Assess heart rate and rhythm
+ Determine heart's electrical axis
+ Examine leads aV$_L$, aV$_F$, and aV$_R$ and R and S waves in precordial leads

ting. Standardization markings are usually located at the beginning of the strip.

5. Assess the heart's rate and rhythm.

6. Determine the heart's electrical axis. Use either the quadrant method or the degree method, which are described later in this chapter.

7. Examine limb leads I, II, and III. The R wave in lead II should be taller than in lead I. The R wave in lead III should be a smaller version of the R wave in lead I. The P wave or QRS complex may be inverted. Each lead should have flat ST segments and upright T waves. Pathologic Q waves should be absent.

8. Examine limb leads aV$_L$, aV$_F$, and aV$_R$. The tracings from leads aV$_L$ and aV$_F$ should be similar, but lead aV$_F$ should have taller P and R waves. Lead aV$_R$ has little diagnostic value. Its P wave, QRS complex, and T wave should be deflected downward.

9. Examine the R wave in the precordial leads. Normally, the R wave — the first positive deflection of the QRS complex — gets progressively taller from lead V$_1$ to V$_5$. It gets slightly smaller in lead V$_6$. (See *R-wave progression*.)

10. Examine the S wave (the negative deflection after an R wave) in the precordial leads. It should appear extremely deep in lead V$_1$ and become progressively more shallow, usually disappearing by lead V$_5$.

Waveform abnormalities

+ Peaked, notched, or enlarged P waves (atrial hypertrophy, enlargement)
+ Inverted P waves (retrograde conduction)
+ Absent P waves (conduction route other than SA node)
+ Short PR intervals (impulses originating somewhere other than SA node)
+ Prolonged PR intervals (conduction delay)
+ Prolonged QRS complex (ventricular conduction)
+ One or more missing QRS complexes (AV block, ventricular standstill)
+ Abnormal Q wave (myocardial necrosis)

WAVEFORM ABNORMALITIES

As you examine each lead, note where changes occur so you can identify the area of the heart affected. Remember that P waves should be upright; however, they may be inverted in lead aV$_R$ or biphasic or inverted in leads III, aV$_L$, and V$_1$. Peaked, notched, or enlarged P waves may signify atrial hypertrophy or enlargement. Inverted P waves may signify retrograde conduction. Absent P waves may signify conduction by a route other than the sinoatrial (SA) node.

PR intervals should always be constant, just like QRS-complex durations. Short PR intervals (less than 0.12 second) signify impulses originating somewhere other than the SA node, as in junctional arrhythmias or preexcitation syndromes. Prolonged PR intervals (greater than 0.20 second) signify a conduction delay, as in heart block or digoxin toxicity.

QRS-complex deflections will vary in different leads. A duration greater than 0.12 second may signify ventricular conduction. One or more missing QRS complexes may signify atrioventricular (AV) block or ventricular standstill. Observe for pathologic Q waves. A normal Q wave generally has a duration of under 0.04 second. An abnormal Q wave has either a duration of 0.04 second or more, a depth greater than 4 mm, or a height one-fourth of the R wave.

R-wave progression

R waves should progress normally through the precordial leads. Note that the R wave in this strip is the first positive deflection in the QRS complex. Also note that the S wave gets smaller, or regresses, from lead V_1 to V_6 until it finally disappears.

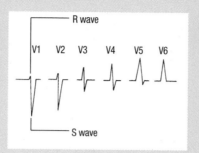

Abnormal Q waves indicate myocardial necrosis. These waves develop when depolarization can't follow its normal path due to damaged tissue in the area. Lead aV_R normally has a large Q wave, so disregard this lead when searching for abnormal Q waves.

 AGE CHANGE Q waves in leads II, III, aV_F, V_5, and V_6 are normal in children. Q waves in other leads suggest cardiac disease such as an abnormal left coronary artery.

ST segments should be isoelectric or have minimal deviation. ST-segment elevation greater than 1 mm above the baseline and ST-segment depression greater than 0.5 mm below the baseline are considered abnormal. Leads facing an injured area will have ST-segment elevations, and leads facing away will show ST-segment depressions.

The T wave normally deflects upward in leads I, II, and V_3 through V_6. It's inverted in lead aV_R and variable in the other leads. Tall, peaked or tented T waves may signify myocardial injury or hyperkalemia. Inverted T waves may signify myocardial ischemia.

A prolonged QT interval (greater than 0.44 second) indicates prolonged ventricular repolarization or congenital prolonged QT syndrome. A short QT interval (less than 0.36 second) may result from digoxin toxicity or hypercalcemia.

ELECTRICAL AXIS

The electrical axis is the average direction of the heart's electrical activity during ventricular depolarization. Leads placed on the body sense the sum of the heart's electrical activity and record it as waveforms.

Waveform abnormalities
(continued)

+ ST segment elevation or depression considered abnormal
+ Tall, peaked, or tented T waves (myocardial injury, hyperkalemia)
+ Inverted T waves (myocardial ischemia)
+ Prolonged QT interval (prolonged ventricular repolarization, congenital prolonged QT syndrome)
+ Short QT interval (digoxin toxicity, hypercalcemia)

Electrical axis
+ Direction of electrical activity during ventricular depolarization

Hexaxial reference system

The hexaxial reference system consists of six bisecting lines, each representing one of the six limb leads, and a circle, representing the heart. The intersection of all lines divides the circle into equal, 30-degree segments.

positive-degree designation doesn't necessarily mean that the pole is positive.

SHIFTING DEGREES
Note that 0 degrees appears at the 3 o'clock position (positive pole lead I). Moving counterclockwise, the degrees become increasingly negative, until reaching ±180 degrees, at the 9 o'clock position (negative pole lead I).
The bottom half of the circle contains the corresponding positive degrees. However, a

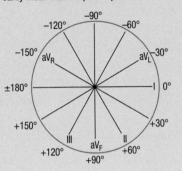

Electrical axis
(continued)

✦ Determined by examining waveforms recorded from six frontal leads (I, II, III, aV_R, aV_L, aV_F)

You can determine your patient's electrical axis by examining the waveforms recorded from the six frontal plane leads: I, II, III, aV_R, aV_L, and aV_F. Imaginary lines drawn from each of the leads intersect at the center of the heart and form a diagram known as the hexaxial reference system. (See *Hexaxial reference system.*)

An axis that falls between 0 and 90 degrees is considered normal (some sources consider –30 to 90 degrees to be normal). An axis between 90 and 180 degrees indicates right axis deviation, and one between 0 and –90 degrees indicates left axis deviation (some sources consider –30 to –90 degrees to be left axis deviation). An axis between –180 and –90 degrees indicates extreme right axis deviation and is called an indeterminate axis.

AGE CHANGE Right axis deviation, between +60 degrees and +160 degrees, is normal in the neonate due to dominance of the right ventricle. By age 1 year, the axis shifts to fall between +10 degrees and +100 degrees as the left ventricle becomes dominant.

Left axis deviation commonly occurs in elderly patients. This axis shift may result from fibrosis of the anterior fascicle of the left bundle branch and because the thickness of the left ventricular wall increases by 25% between ages 30 and 80.

Electrical axis determination

✦ Quadrant or degree method

ELECTRICAL AXIS DETERMINATION

To determine your patient's electrical axis, use the quadrant method or the degree method.

Quadrant method

The quadrant method, a fast, easy way to plot the heart's axis, involves observing the main deflection of the QRS complex in leads I and aV$_F$. (See *Quadrant method*.) Lead I indicates whether impulses are moving to the right or left, and lead aV$_F$ indicates whether they're moving up or down.

If the QRS-complex deflection is positive or upright in both leads, the electrical axis is normal. If lead I is upright and lead aV$_F$ points down, left axis deviation exists.

When lead I points down and lead aV$_F$ is upright, right axis deviation exists. Both waves pointing down signal extreme right axis deviation.

Degree method

A more precise axis calculation, the degree method provides an exact measurement of the electrical axis. (See *Degree method*, page 214.) It also allows

Quadrant method

✦ Observe main deflection of QRS complex in leads I and aV$_F$
✦ Lead I shows whether impulses are moving to right or left
✦ Lead aV$_F$ shows whether they're moving up or down
✦ If QRS-complex deflection positive or upright in both, axis is normal

Degree method

✦ Provides a more exact measurement of electrical axis

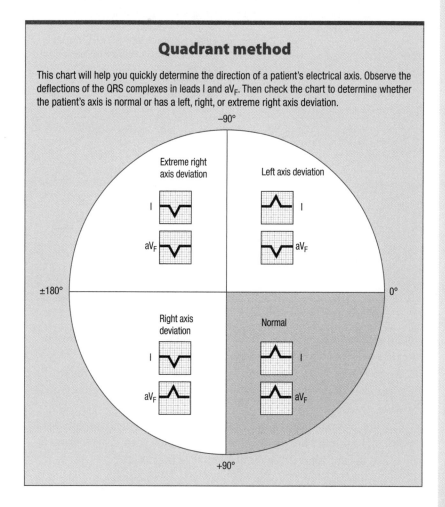

Quadrant method

This chart will help you quickly determine the direction of a patient's electrical axis. Observe the deflections of the QRS complexes in leads I and aV$_F$. Then check the chart to determine whether the patient's axis is normal or has a left, right, or extreme right axis deviation.

Degree method

The degree method of determining axis deviation allows you to identify a patient's electrical axis by degrees on the hexaxial system, not just by quadrant. To use this method, take the following steps.

STEP 1
Identify the limb lead with the smallest QRS complex or the equiphasic QRS complex. In this example, it's lead III.

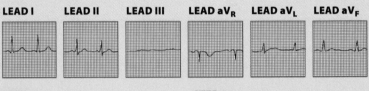

LEAD I   **LEAD II**   **LEAD III**   **LEAD aV$_R$**   **LEAD aV$_L$**   **LEAD aV$_F$**

STEP 2
Locate the axis for lead III on the hexaxial diagram. Then find the axis perpendicular to it, which is the axis for lead aV$_R$.

STEP 3
Now, examine the QRS complex in lead aV$_R$, noting whether the deflection is positive or negative. As you can see, the QRS complex for this lead is negative, indicating that the current is moving toward the negative pole of aV$_R$, which is in the right lower quadrant at +30 degrees on the hexaxial diagram. So the electrical axis here is normal at +30 degrees.

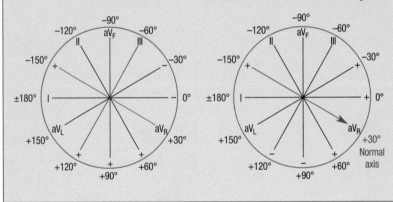

Degree method
(continued)
+ Identify lead containing smallest QRS complex or complex with equal deflection
+ Use hexaxial diagram to find lead perpendicular to this lead; examine its QRS complex
+ Plot this on hexaxial diagram to determine electrical axis direction

you to determine the axis even if the QRS complex isn't clearly positive or negative in leads I and aV$_F$. To use this method, follow these steps.

1. Review all six leads, and identify the one that contains either the smallest QRS complex or the complex with an equal deflection above and below the baseline.

2. Use the hexaxial diagram to identify the lead perpendicular to this lead. For example, if lead I has the smallest QRS complex, then the lead perpendicular to the line representing lead I would be lead aV$_F$.

3. After you've identified the perpendicular lead, examine its QRS complex. If the electrical activity is moving toward the positive pole of a lead, the QRS complex deflects upward. If it's moving away from the positive pole of a lead, the QRS complex deflects downward.

4. Plot this information on the hexaxial diagram to determine the direction of the electrical axis.

Axis deviation

Finding a patient's electrical axis can help confirm a diagnosis or narrow the range of possible diagnoses. Factors that influence the location of the axis include the heart's position in the chest, the heart's size, the patient's body size or type, the conduction pathways, and the force of the electrical impulses being generated. Causes of left axis deviation include:

✦ normal variation
✦ inferior wall myocardial infarction (MI)
✦ left anterior hemiblock
✦ Wolff-Parkinson-White (WPW) syndrome
✦ mechanical shifts (ascites, pregnancy, tumors)
✦ left bundle-branch block (LBBB)
✦ left ventricular hypertrophy (LVH)
✦ aortic stenosis
✦ aging.
   Causes of right axis deviation include:
✦ normal variation
✦ lateral wall MI
✦ left posterior hemiblock
✦ right bundle-branch block (RBBB)
✦ emphysema
✦ right ventricular hypertrophy
✦ pulmonary hypertension
✦ pulmonic stenosis.

   Remember that electrical activity in the heart swings away from areas of damage or necrosis, so the damaged part of the heart will be the last area depolarized. For example, in RBBB, the impulse travels quickly down the normal left side and then moves slowly down the right side. This shifts the electrical forces to the right, causing right axis deviation.

   Axis deviation isn't always clinically significant, and it isn't always cardiac in origin. For example, infants and children normally have right axis deviation. Pregnant women normally have left axis deviation.

Axis deviation

✦ Helps confirm a diagnosis
✦ Electrical activity moves away from damage or necrosis; damaged part last area depolarized

Causes of left axis deviation

✦ Normal variation
✦ inferior wall MI
✦ LAH
✦ WPW syndrome
✦ Mechanical shifts
✦ LBBB
✦ LVH
✦ Aortic stenosis
✦ Aging

Causes of right axis deviation

✦ Normal variation
✦ Lateral wall MI
✦ Left posterior hemiblock
✦ RBBB
✦ Emphysema
✦ RVH
✦ Pulmonary hypertension
✦ Pulmonary stenosis

DISORDERS AFFECTING 12-LEAD ECGS

A 12-lead ECG is used to assist in the diagnosis of certain conditions such as angina, Prinzmetal's angina, myocardial infarction, pericarditis, left ventricular hypertrophy, and bundle-branch block. By reviewing sample ECGs, you'll know the classic signs to look for. This section examines ECG characteristics of each of these cardiac conditions.

Angina

+ Myocardium requires more oxygen than coronary arteries can supply

Causes

+ Arteries narrowing from CAD; may be complicated by platelet clumping, thrombus formation, and vasospasm

Signs and symptoms

+ Most patients with either *stable* or *unstable* angina show ischemic changes on ECG only during attack

Stable angina
+ Substernal pain or precordial burning, squeezing, or tightness
+ May radiate to left arm, neck, or jaw
+ Perhaps triggered by exertion or stress; usually relieved by rest

Unstable angina
+ More easily provoked, commonly waking patient
+ Unpredictable, worsening over time
+ Treated as medical emergency

ANGINA

During an episode of angina, the myocardium demands more oxygen than the coronary arteries can deliver. An episode of angina usually lasts between 2 and 10 minutes. The closer to 30 minutes the pain lasts, the more likely it's from myocardial infarction (MI) rather than angina.

Angina is classified as an acute coronary syndrome. The term stable angina has been applied to certain conditions and unstable angina applied to others.

CAUSES

Decreased blood flow results from narrowing of the arteries from coronary artery disease (CAD), which may be complicated by platelet clumping, thrombus formation, and vasospasm.

SIGNS AND SYMPTOMS

In stable angina, pain is substernal or precordial burning, squeezing, or tightness and may radiate to the left arm, neck, or jaw. It may be triggered by exertion or stress and is typically relieved by rest. Each episode follows the same pattern.

Unstable angina, on the other hand, is more easily provoked, commonly waking the patient. Chest pain may not radiate and is of greater intensity and duration than in stable angina. It's also unpredictable and worsens over time. The patient's skin may be pale and clammy and he may feel nauseous and anxious. Unstable angina is treated as a medical emergency because its onset usually portends an MI.

Most patients with either form of angina show ischemic changes on an ECG only during the attack. (See *ECG changes associated with angina.*) Because these changes may be fleeting, always obtain an order for, and perform, a 12-lead ECG as soon as the patient reports chest pain.

The ECG will help you determine which area of the heart and which coronary arteries are involved. By recognizing danger early, you may be able to prevent MI or even death.

ECG changes associated with angina

Illustrated below are some classic ECG changes involving the T wave and ST segment that you may see when monitoring a patient with angina.

PEAKED T WAVE	**FLATTENED T WAVE**	**T-WAVE INVERSION**	**ST-SEGMENT DEPRESSION WITH T-WAVE INVERSION**	**ST-SEGMENT DEPRESSION WITHOUT T-WAVE INVERSION**

INTERVENTIONS

Drugs are a key component of treating angina. Nitrates are given to reduce myocardial oxygen consumption. Beta-adrenergic blockers are used to reduce the heart's workload and oxygen demands. Calcium channel blockers treat angina caused by coronary vasospasm. Antiplatelet drugs are used to minimize platelet aggregation and the risk of coronary occlusion. Antilipemic drugs reduce elevated serum cholesterol or triglycerides levels. If the patient has continued unstable angina or acute chest pain give glycoprotein IIb/IIIa inhibitors to reduce platelet aggregation. Anticipate coronary artery bypass surgery or percutaneous transluminal coronary angioplasty for obstructive lesions.

PRINZMETAL'S ANGINA

Prinzmetal's angina is a relatively uncommon form of unstable angina. Ischemic pain usually occurs at rest or awakens the patient from sleep. Pain doesn't follow physical activity or emotional stress.

CAUSES

Prinzmetal's angina is caused by a focal episodic spasm of a coronary artery, with or without the presence of an obstructing coronary artery lesion.

Interventions
+ Nitrates reduce myocardial oxygen consumption
+ Beta-adrenergic blockers reduce heart's workload and oxygen demands
+ Calcium channel blockers treat angina caused by coronary vasospasm
+ Antiplatelet drugs minimize platelet aggregation and risk of coronary occlusion
+ Antilipemic drugs reduce serum cholesterol or triglyceride levels

Prinzmetal's angina
+ Uncommon form of unstable angina
+ Ischemic pain occurs at rest or awakens patient

Causes
+ Focal episodic coronary artery spasm

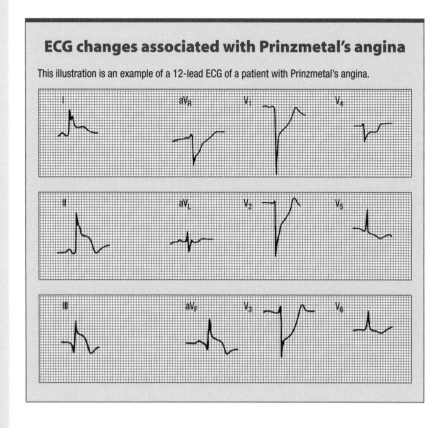

ECG changes associated with Prinzmetal's angina

This illustration is an example of a 12-lead ECG of a patient with Prinzmetal's angina.

ECG characteristics

+ *ST segment*—elevation in leads monitoring area of coronary spasm; occurs with chest pain, resolves when it subsides

ECG CHARACTERISTICS

Rhythm: Atrial and ventricular rhythms are normal.

Rate: Atrial and ventricular rates are within normal limits.

P wave: Normal size and configuration.

PR interval: Normal.

QRS complex: Normal.

ST segment: Marked elevation in leads monitoring the heart area where the coronary spasm occurs. This elevation occurs during chest pain and resolves when pain subsides. (See *ECG changes associated with Prinzmetal's angina.*)

T wave: Usually of normal size and configuration.

QT interval: Normal.

Other: None.

Signs and symptoms

+ Substernal chest pain, ranging from heavy feeling to crushing discomfort (usually at rest)

SIGNS AND SYMPTOMS

A patient with Prinzmetal's angina typically experiences substernal chest pain ranging from a feeling of heaviness to a crushing discomfort, usually while at rest. He may also experience dyspnea, nausea, vomiting, diaphoresis, and arrhythmias.

INTERVENTIONS

Acute management includes the administration of nitroglycerin, which should provide prompt relief from pain by dilating the coronary arteries. For chronic management, long-acting nitrates and calcium channel blockers may be used to help prevent coronary artery spasm. Patients with obstructing coronary artery lesions may benefit from revascularization.

MYOCARDIAL INFARCTION

Myocardial infarction (MI) is categorized as an acute coronary syndrome. Reduced blood flow through one or more coronary arteries causes myocardial ischemia, injury, and necrosis. Damage usually occurs in the left ventricle, although the location varies depending on the coronary artery affected. For as long as the myocardium is deprived of an oxygen-rich blood supply, an ECG will reflect the three pathologic changes of an MI: ischemia, injury, and infarction. (See *Reciprocal changes in MI,* page 220.)

CAUSES

Causes of MI include atherosclerosis and embolus. In atherosclerosis, plaque (an unstable and lipid-rich substance) forms and subsequently ruptures or erodes, resulting in platelet adhesions, fibrin clot formation, and activation of thrombin.

   Risk factors for MI include:
+ diabetes
+ family history of heart disease
+ high-fat, high-carbohydrate diet
+ hyperlipoproteinemia
+ hypertension
+ menopause
+ obesity
+ sedentary lifestyle
+ smoking
+ stress.

ECG CHARACTERISTICS

The area of myocardial necrosis is called the zone of infarction. Scar tissue eventually replaces the dead tissue, and the damage caused is irreversible. The cardinal ECG change associated with a necrotic area is a pathologic Q wave, which results from lack of depolarization. Such Q waves are permanent. MIs that don't produce Q waves are called non–Q-wave MIs.

Interventions
+ *Acute* — Nitroglycerin provides prompt relief by dilating coronary arteries
+ *Chronic* — Long-acting nitrates and calcium channel blockers prevent coronary artery spasm

MI
+ Classified as acute coronary syndrome
+ Reduced blood flow through one or more coronary arteries causes myocardial ischemia, injury, and necrosis

Causes
+ Atherosclerosis and embolus

Risk factors
+ Diabetes
+ Family history of heart disease
+ High-fat, high-carbohydrate diet
+ Hyperlipoproteinemia
+ Hypertension
+ Menopause
+ Obesity
+ Sedentary lifestyle
+ Smoking
+ Stress

ECG characteristics
+ Cardinal ECG change associated with necrotic area is pathologic Q wave

Reciprocal changes in MI

Ischemia, injury, and infarction — the three Is of myocardial infarction (MI) — produce characteristic ECG changes. The changes shown by leads that reflect electrical activity in damaged areas are shown on the right of the illustration below.

Reciprocal leads, those opposite the damaged area, show opposing ECG changes, as shown to the left of the illustration.

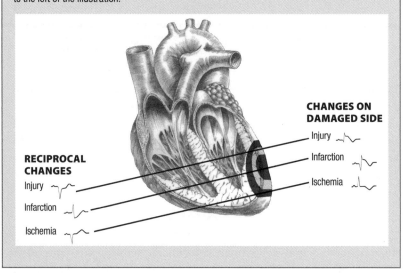

CHANGES ON DAMAGED SIDE
Injury
Infarction
Ischemia

RECIPROCAL CHANGES
Injury
Infarction
Ischemia

ECG characteristics
(continued)

✦ *Non–Q-wave MI* —non–ST-segment elevation or ST-segment depression
✦ *Q-wave MI* —ST-segment elevation and Q waves (representing scarring, necrosis)
✦ *Elevated ST segment* —zone of injury
✦ *T-wave inversion* —zone of ischemia
✦ ST segments return to baseline within 2 weeks; T waves may persist for several months
✦ Q waves that do appear remain indefinitely

✦ In a non–Q-wave MI, abnormalities may include non–ST-segment elevation or ST-segment depression.

✦ In a Q-wave MI, abnormalities may include ST-segment elevation and Q waves, which represent scarring and necrosis.

The zone of infarction is surrounded by the zone of injury, which appears on an ECG as an elevated ST segment. ST-segment elevation results from a prolonged lack of blood supply.

The outermost area of the zone of infarction is called the zone of ischemia and results from an interrupted blood supply. This zone is represented on an ECG by T-wave inversion. Changes in the zones of ischemia or injury are reversible.

Generally, as an MI occurs, the patient experiences chest pain, and an ECG will display such changes as ST-segment elevation, which indicates that myocardial injury is occurring. T waves generally flatten and eventually invert.

Rapid treatment can prevent myocardial necrosis. However, if symptoms persist for more than 6 hours, little can be done to prevent necrosis. That's one of the reasons patients are advised to seek medical attention as soon as symptoms begin.

Knowing how long such changes last can help you determine how long ago an MI occurred. After the first few days, ST segments return to baseline within 2 weeks. Inverted T waves may persist for several months. Although Q waves don't appear on the ECG of every patient who suffers an MI, when the waves do appear, they remain indefinitely.

SIGNS AND SYMPTOMS

Signs and symptoms of an MI may include:
+ chest pain:
– severe, persistent, burning, squeezing, or crushing
– usually substernal or precordial
– may radiate to left arm, neck, jaw, or shoulder blade
– lasts at least 20 minutes and may persist for several hours
– unrelieved by rest.
+ other signs and symptoms:
– anxiety
– cool extremities
– fatigue
– feeling of impending doom
– hypertension
– hypotension
– nausea
– shortness of breath
– vomiting.
+ atypical presentation:
– more likely in women, elderly patients, and patients with diabetes
– may include vague or absent chest discomfort; jaw, back, or shoulder pain; shortness of breath; fatigue; or abdominal discomfort.

INTERVENTIONS

If a patient develops chest pain, take immediate measures to decrease cardiac workload and increase oxygen supply to the myocardium. These measures include rest, pain relief, and supplemental oxygen.
+ If symptoms started during previous 3 hours, prepare for thrombolytic therapy (unless contraindicated) to restore vessel patency and minimize necrosis.
+ Give oxygen to increase oxygenation of blood.
+ Give nitroglycerin sublingually to relieve chest pain (unless systolic blood pressure is less than 90 mm Hg or heart rate is less than 50 or more than 100 beats/minute).
+ Give morphine to relieve pain.
+ Give aspirin to inhibit platelet aggregation.

Signs and symptoms

Chest pain
+ Severe, persistent, burning, squeezing, or crushing
+ Substernal or precordial (usually)
+ May radiate to left arm, neck, jaw, or shoulder blade
+ Duration at least 20 minutes, perhaps several hours
+ Unrelieved by rest

Other signs and symptoms
+ Anxiety
+ Cool extremities
+ Fatigue
+ Feeling of impending doom
+ Hypertension, hypotension
+ Nausea, vomiting
+ Shortness of breath

Atypical presentation
+ More likely in women, elderly patients, and patients with diabetes

Interventions
+ Prepare for thrombolytic therapy, if symptoms started within previous 3 hours
+ Give oxygen to increase oxygenation
+ Give nitroglycerin for chest pain
+ Give morphine for pain
+ Give aspirin to inhibit platelet aggregation

Interventions
(continued)

+ Give I.V. heparin if patient received tissue plasminogen activator
+ Give antiarrhythmics if patient has arrhythmia
+ Give glycoprotein IIb/IIIa inhibitors to reduce platelet aggregation
+ Prepare patient for interventional or surgical procedures

+ If the patient received tissue plasminogen activator, give I.V. heparin to promote patency in the affected coronary artery.

+ If the patient has arrhythmia, prepare for use of antiarrhythmics, transcutaneous pacing patches (or transvenous pacemaker), defibrillation, or epinephrine.

+ A patient without hypotension, bradycardia, or excessive tachycardia may receive I.V. nitroglycerin for 24 to 48 hours to reduce afterload and preload and relieve chest pain.

+ If the patient has continued unstable angina or acute chest pain or has had an invasive cardiac procedure, give glycoprotein IIb/IIIa inhibitors to reduce platelet aggregation.

+ Interventional procedures, such as percutaneous transluminal angioplasty, stent placement, or coronary artery atherectomy; or surgical procedures such as coronary artery bypass graft may open blocked or narrowed arteries.

Types of MI

+ Location critical factor in planning treatment and predicting complications

TYPES OF MYOCARDIAL INFARCTION

The location of the myocardial infarction (MI) is a critical factor in determining the most appropriate treatment and predicting probable complications. Characteristic ECG changes that occur with each type of MI are localized to the leads overlying the infarction site. (See *Locating myocardial damage.*) This section takes a look at characteristic ECG changes that occur with different types of MIs.

Anterior wall MI

+ Left anterior descending artery becomes occluded
+ Changes appear in leads V_2 to V_4

ANTERIOR WALL MI

The left anterior descending artery supplies blood to the anterior portion of the left ventricle, ventricular septum, and portions of the right and left bundle-branch systems.

When the left anterior descending artery becomes occluded, an anterior wall MI occurs. (See *Recognizing an anterior wall MI,* page 224.) Complications include second-degree AV blocks, bundle-branch blocks, ventricular irritability, and left-sided heart failure.

An anterior wall MI causes characteristic ECG changes in leads V_2 to V_4. The precordial leads show poor R-wave progression because the left ventricle can't depolarize normally. ST-segment elevation and T-wave inversion are also present.

The reciprocal leads for the anterior wall are the inferior leads II, III, and aV_F. They initially show tall R waves and depressed ST segments.

Locating myocardial damage

After you've noted characteristic lead changes in an acute myocardial infarction, use this table to identify the areas of damage. Match the lead changes (ST elevation, abnormal Q waves) in the second column with the affected wall in the first column and the artery involved in the third column. The fourth column shows reciprocal lead changes.

WALL AFFECTED	LEADS	ARTERY INVOLVED	RECIPROCAL CHANGES
Anterior	V_2, V_3, V_4	Left coronary artery, left anterior descending (LAD)	II, III, aV_F
Anterolateral	I, aV_L, V_3, V_4, V_5, V_6	LAD and diagonal branches, circumflex and marginal branches	II, III, aV_F
Anteroseptal	V_1, V_2, V_3, V_4	LAD	None
Inferior	II, III, aV_F	Right coronary artery (RCA)	I, aV_L
Lateral	I, aV_L, V_5, V_6	Circumflex branch of left coronary artery	II, III, aV_F
Posterior	V_8, V_9	RCA or circumflex	V_1, V_2, V_3, V_4 (R greater than S in V_1 and V_2, ST-segment depression, elevated T wave)
Right ventricular	V_{4R}, V_{5R}, V_{6R}	RCA	None

SEPTAL WALL MI

The patient with a septal wall MI is at increased risk for developing a ventricular septal defect. ECG changes are present in leads V_1 and V_2. In those leads, the R wave disappears, the ST segment rises, and the T wave inverts. Because the left anterior descending artery also supplies blood to the ventricular septum, a septal wall MI typically accompanies an anterior wall MI.

LATERAL WALL MI

A lateral wall MI is usually caused by a blockage in the left circumflex artery and shows characteristic changes in the left lateral leads I, aV_L, V_5, and V_6. The reciprocal leads for a lateral wall infarction are leads V_1 and V_2. (See *Recognizing a lateral wall MI*, page 225.)

Septal wall MI
+ Patient at increased risk for ventricular septal defect
+ Changes appear in leads V_1 and V_2

Lateral wall MI
+ Blockage in left circumflex artery
+ Changes appear in left lateral leads I, aV_L, V_5, and V_6

Recognizing an anterior wall MI

This 12-lead ECG shows typical characteristics of an anterior wall myocardial infarction (MI). Note that the R waves don't progress through the precordial leads. Also note the ST-segment elevation in leads V_2 and V_3. As expected, the reciprocal leads II, III, and aV_F show slight ST-segment depression. Axis deviation is normal at +60 degrees.

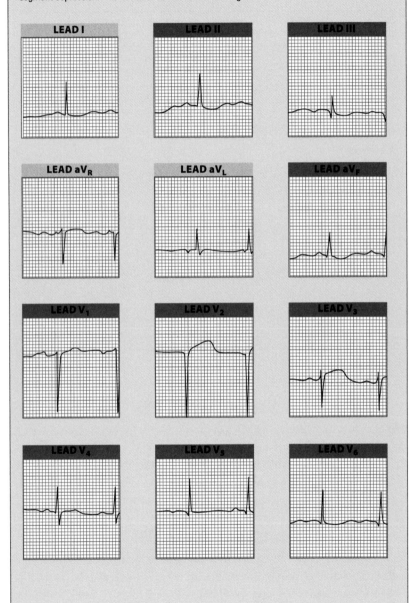

Recognizing a lateral wall MI

This 12-lead ECG shows typical characteristics of a lateral wall myocardial infarction (MI). Note the ST-segment elevation in leads I, aV$_L$, V$_5$, and V$_6$.

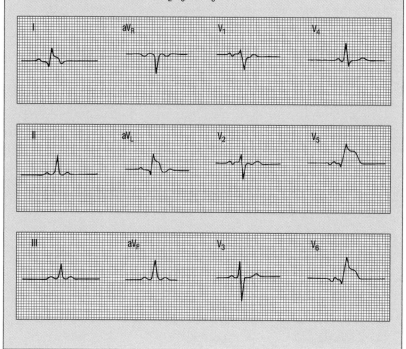

A lateral wall MI typically causes premature ventricular contractions (PVCs) and varying degrees of heart block. It usually accompanies an anterior or inferior wall MI.

INFERIOR WALL MI

An inferior wall MI is usually caused by occlusion of the right coronary artery and produces characteristic ECG changes in the inferior leads II, III, and aV$_F$ and reciprocal changes in the lateral leads I and aV$_L$. (See *Recognizing an inferior wall MI,* page 226.) It's also called a diaphragmatic MI because the inferior wall of the heart lies over the diaphragm.

Patients with inferior wall MI are at risk for developing sinus bradycardia, sinus arrest, heart block, and PVCs. This type of MI occurs alone or with a lateral wall or right ventricular MI.

Inferior wall MI
✦ Occlusion of right coronary artery
✦ Changes appear in inferior leads II, III, and aV$_F$

Recognizing an inferior wall MI

This 12-lead ECG shows the characteristic changes of an inferior wall myocardial infarction (MI). In leads II, III, and aV$_F$, note the T-wave inversion, ST-segment elevation, and pathologic Q waves. In leads I and aV$_L$, note the slight ST-segment depression — a reciprocal change. This ECG shows left axis deviation at –60 degrees.

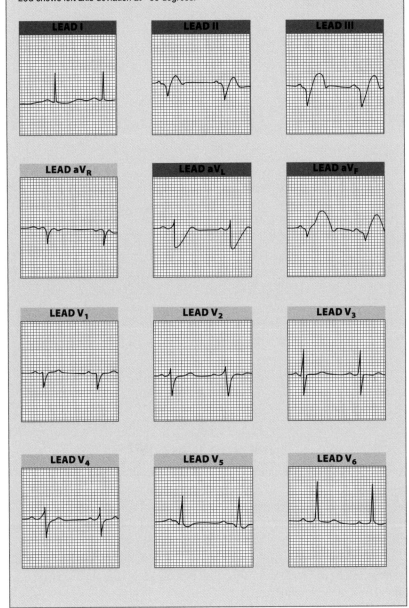

Recognizing a right ventricular MI

This 12-lead ECG shows typical characteristics of a right ventricular myocardial infarction (MI). Note the ST-segment elevation in the right precordial chest leads V_{4R}, V_{5R}, and V_{6R}. Pathologic Q waves would also appear in leads V_{4R}, V_{5R}, and V_{6R}.

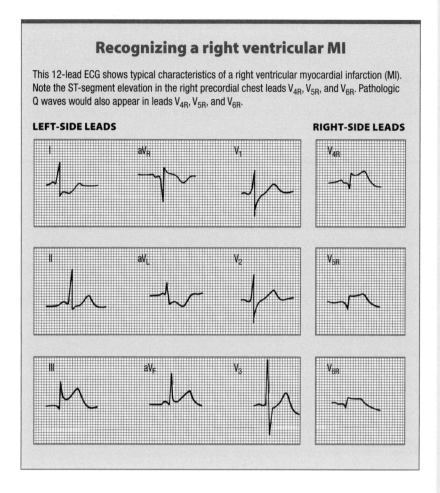

LEFT-SIDE LEADS

RIGHT-SIDE LEADS

POSTERIOR WALL MI

A posterior wall MI is caused by occlusion of the right coronary artery or the left circumflex arteries. It produces reciprocal changes in leads V_1 to V_4.

ECG changes for a posterior wall MI include tall R waves, ST-segment depression, and upright T waves. Posterior infarctions may accompany inferior infarctions. Data about the posterior wall and pathologic Q waves that might occur can be obtained from leads V_8 and V_9, using a posterior ECG.

RIGHT VENTRICULAR MI

A right ventricular MI usually follows occlusion of the right coronary artery. This type of MI rarely occurs alone. In 40% of patients, a right ventricular MI accompanies an inferior wall MI. (See *Recognizing a right ventricular MI.*)

Posterior wall MI

+ Occlusion of right coronary artery or left circumflex arteries
+ Reciprocal changes appear in leads V_1 to V_4

Right ventricular MI

+ Usually follows occlusion of right coronary artery
+ Changes appear as ST-segment elevation, pathologic Q waves, and inverted T waves in right precordial leads V_{2R} to V_{6R}

A right ventricular MI can lead to right ventricular failure. The classic changes are ST-segment elevation, pathologic Q waves, and inverted T waves in the right precordial leads V_{2R} to V_{6R}. Identifying a right ventricular MI is difficult without information from the right precordial leads. If these leads aren't available, you can observe leads II, III, and aV_F or watch leads V_1, V_2, and V_3 for ST-segment elevation. If a right ventricular MI has occurred, use lead II to monitor for further damage.

Pericarditis

+ Inflammation of pericardium; either acute or chronic

Causes

+ Viral, bacterial, or fungal disorders
+ Rheumatic fever
+ Autoimmune disorders
+ Complications of cardiac injury

ECG characteristics

+ In earliest stage, elevations in ST segments accompany upright T waves
+ In second stage, ST segment resolves, with widespread T-wave inversion
+ ST-segment elevation main abnormality and usually appears in most (if not all) leads, except aV_R

PERICARDITIS

Pericarditis is an inflammation of the pericardium, the fibroserous sac that envelops the heart. Pericarditis can be either acute or chronic. The acute form may be fibrinous or effusive, with purulent, serous, or hemorrhagic exudate. Chronic constrictive pericarditis causes dense fibrous thickening of the pericardium.

CAUSES

Possible causes of pericarditis include:

+ viral, bacterial, or fungal disorders
+ rheumatic fever
+ autoimmune disorders
+ complications of cardiac injury (myocardial infarction [MI], cardiotomy).

Regardless of the form, pericarditis can cause cardiac tamponade if fluid accumulates too quickly. It can also cause heart failure if constriction occurs.

ECG CHARACTERISTICS

In pericarditis, ECG changes occur in four stages of disease progression. These changes are secondary to myocardial inflammation and excessive pericardial fluid or a thickened pericardium.

ECG changes evolve through two stages. In the earliest stage, elevation of ST segments accompanies upright T waves. Typically, resolution of the ST-segment elevation marks the beginning of the second stage of acute pericarditis, with widespread T-wave inversion.

The primary ECG abnormality in acute pericarditis is ST-segment elevation. In contrast to the convex ST-segment elevation in acute MI, the ST segments appear somewhat concave in pericarditis. Because pericarditis usually affects the entire myocardial surface, ST segments are usually elevated in most — if not all — leads, except lead aV_R. (See *Comparing MI with acute pericarditis.*)

Rhythm: Atrial and ventricular rhythms are usually regular.

Comparing MI with acute pericarditis

Myocardial infarction (MI) and acute pericarditis cause ST-segment elevation on an ECG. However, the ST segment and T wave (shaded areas) on an MI waveform are quite different from those on the pericarditis waveform.

In addition, because pericarditis involves the surrounding pericardium, several leads will show ST-segment and T-wave changes (typically leads I, II, aV$_F$, and V$_4$ through V$_6$). In MI, however, only those leads reflecting the area of infarction will show the characteristic changes.

These rhythm strips demonstrate the ECG variations between MI and acute pericarditis.

MYOCARDIAL INFARCTION

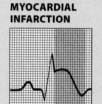

ACUTE PERICARDITIS

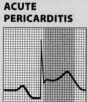

Rate: Atrial and ventricular rates usually remain within normal limits.

P wave: Normal size and configuration.

PR interval: Usually normal.

QRS complex: Normal, but a possible decrease in amplitude may occur.

ST segment: In stage 1, the ST segment is elevated 1 to 2 mm in leads II, III, and aV$_F$ as well as in the precordial leads.

T wave: Remains elevated during the acute phase of pericarditis. As the pericarditis resolves, the T waves become inverted in the leads that had the ST-segment elevation.

QT interval: Normal.

Other: Atrial fibrillation, atrial flutter, or tachycardia may occur as a result of sinoatrial node irritation.

SIGNS AND SYMPTOMS

A patient with acute pericarditis may complain of chest pain, dyspnea, and chills. He may experience fever, diaphoresis, and arrhythmias. A pericardial friction rub is commonly heard. The chest pain typically worsens with deep inspiration and improves when the patient sits up and leans forward.

A patient with chronic pericarditis usually experiences symptoms similar to chronic right-sided heart failure, including edema, ascites, and hepatomegaly.

The most distinctive clinical feature is a palpable, and sometimes audible, sharp knock or rub in early diastole, when the rapidly filling ventricle touches the unexpansive pericardium.

ECG characteristics
(continued)

✦ *ST segment*—in stage 1, elevated 1 to 2 mm in leads II, III, and aV$_F$ and in precordial leads

✦ *T wave*—elevated during acute phase; with resolution, inverted in leads that had ST-segment elevation

Signs and symptoms

Acute pericarditis
✦ Chest pain
✦ Dyspnea
✦ Chills
✦ Fever
✦ Diaphoresis
✦ Arrhythmias

Chronic pericarditis
✦ Edema
✦ Ascites
✦ Hepatomegaly

Interventions

+ Bed rest and corticosteroids or NSAIDs for acute pericarditis
+ Antibiotics for infectious pericarditis
+ Pericardiocentesis for cardiac tamponade
+ Complete pericardectomy for constrictive pericarditis

LVH

+ Left ventricular wall thickening

Causes

+ Mitral insufficiency
+ Cardiomyopathy
+ Aortic stenosis or insufficiency
+ Systemic hypertension

ECG characteristics

+ *QRS complex*—prolonged or widened with increased amplitude
+ *ST segment*—possibly depressed in precordial leads if associated with T-wave inversion
+ *T wave*—possibly inverted in leads V_5 and V_6 (depending on extent of hypertrophy)
+ *Other*—axis usually normal; left axis deviation may be present

INTERVENTIONS

Acute pericarditis is treated with bed rest and corticosteroids or nonsteroidal anti-inflammatory drugs (NSAIDs) to relieve pain and inflammation. Infectious pericarditis is treated with antibiotics. Pericardiocentesis is performed for cardiac tamponade, and a complete pericardectomy may be performed for constrictive pericarditis. Keep in mind that the underlying cause of the pericarditis needs to be identified and treated.

LEFT VENTRICULAR HYPERTROPHY

In left ventricular hypertrophy (LVH), the left ventricular wall thickens. LVH usually results from conditions that cause chronic increases in pressures within the ventricle.

CAUSES

LVH may be caused by mitral insufficiency, cardiomyopathy, aortic stenosis or insufficiency, or systemic hypertension (the most common cause). LVH may lead to left-sided heart failure, which subsequently leads to increased left atrial pressure, pulmonary vascular congestion, and pulmonary arterial hypertension. LVH can decrease coronary artery perfusion, causing MI, or it can alter the papillary muscle, causing mitral insufficiency.

ECG CHARACTERISTICS

Rhythm: Atrial and ventricular rhythms are normal.
Rate: Atrial and ventricular rates are normal.
P wave: May be normal in size and configuration, or may reflect left atrial enlargement.
PR interval: Normal.
QRS complex: May be prolonged or widened with increased amplitude. In lead I, the R wave's amplitude exceeds 1.4 mV. In leads V_1 and V_2, deeper S waves appear. The sum of the S wave in lead V_1 or V_2 and the R wave in lead V_5 or V_6 exceeds 3.5 mV. The R wave is taller in lead V_6 than in V_5. The R wave's amplitude in lead V_5 or V_6 exceeds 2.6 mV. (See *Recognizing LVH.*)
ST segment: Possibly depressed in the precordial leads when associated with T-wave inversion. This pattern is known as LVH with strain.
T wave: May be inverted in leads V_5 and V_6, depending on the degree of hypertrophy.
QT interval: Usually normal.
Other: The axis is usually normal, but left axis deviation may be present.

Recognizing LVH

Left ventricular hypertrophy (LVH) can lead to heart failure or myocardial infarction. The rhythm strip shown here illustrates key ECG changes of LVH as they occur in selected leads: a large S wave (shaded area below left) in V_1 and a large R wave (shaded area below right) in V_5. If the depth (in mm) of the S wave in V_1 added to the height (in mm) of the R wave in V_5 is greater than 35 mm, then LVH is present.

LEAD V₁

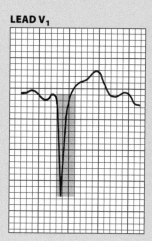

LEAD V₅

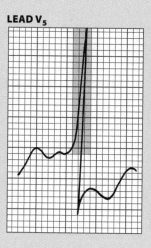

SIGNS AND SYMPTOMS

Signs and symptoms are related to the underlying disorder.

INTERVENTIONS

Interventions are focused on the management of the underlying disorder such as hypertension.

BUNDLE-BRANCH BLOCK

One potential complication of a myocardial infarction (MI) is bundle-branch block (BBB). In this disorder, either the left or the right bundle branch fails to conduct impulses normally. A BBB that occurs toward the distal end of the left bundle, in the posterior or anterior fasciculus, is called a *hemiblock*. Some blocks require treatment with a temporary pacemaker. Others are monitored only to detect whether they progress to a more complete block.

Signs and symptoms
+ Related to underlying disorder

Interventions
+ Identify and treat underlying disorder

BBB
+ Left or right bundle branch fails to conduct impulses normally

BBB
(continued)
+ Impulse travels down unaffected bundle branch, depolarizing ventricle
+ Conduction progresses slowly, so ventricular depolarization is prolonged
+ QRS complex is widened to more than 0.12 second

RBBB
+ Occurs with anterior wall MI, CAD, and pulmonary embolism, but may occur on its own
+ QRS complex > 0.12 second and has different configuration

Lead V$_1$
+ Small R wave remains as septal depolarization unaffected
+ R wave then S wave (left ventricular depolarization) and tall R wave (late right ventricular depolarization)
+ T wave negative

In a BBB, the impulse travels down the unaffected bundle branch and then from one myocardial cell to the next to depolarize the ventricle. Because this cell-to-cell conduction progresses much more slowly than along the specialized cells of the conduction system, ventricular depolarization is prolonged.

Prolonged ventricular depolarization means that the QRS complex widens. The normal width is 0.06 to 0.10 second. If it increases to more than 0.12 second, BBB is present.

After identifying BBB, examine lead V$_1$ and lead V$_6$. You'll use these leads to determine whether the block is in the right or the left bundle branch.

RIGHT BUNDLE-BRANCH BLOCK

Right bundle-branch block (RBBB) occurs with such conditions as anterior wall MI, coronary artery disease (CAD), and pulmonary embolism. It may also occur without cardiac disease. If it develops as heart rate increases, it's called rate-related RBBB. (See *Understanding RBBB.*)

In this disorder, the QRS complex is greater than 0.12 second and has a different configuration, sometimes resembling rabbit ears or the letter "M." (See *Recognizing RBBB.*) Septal depolarization isn't affected in lead V$_1$, so the initial small R wave remains.

The R wave is followed by an S wave, which represents left ventricular depolarization, and a tall R wave (called R prime, or R'), which represents late right ventricular depolarization. The T wave is negative in this lead; however,

Understanding RBBB

In right bundle-branch block (RBBB), the initial impulse activates the interventricular septum from left to right, just as in normal activation (arrow 1). Next, the left bundle branch activates the left ventricle (arrow 2). The impulse then crosses the interventricular septum to activate the right ventricle (arrow 3).

Block

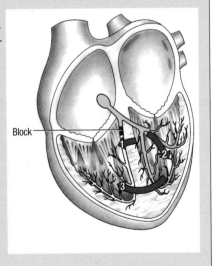

Recognizing RBBB

This 12-lead ECG shows the characteristic changes of right bundle-branch block (RBBB). In lead V_1, note the rsR' pattern and T-wave inversion. In lead V_6, see the widened S wave and the upright T wave. Also note the prolonged QRS complexes.

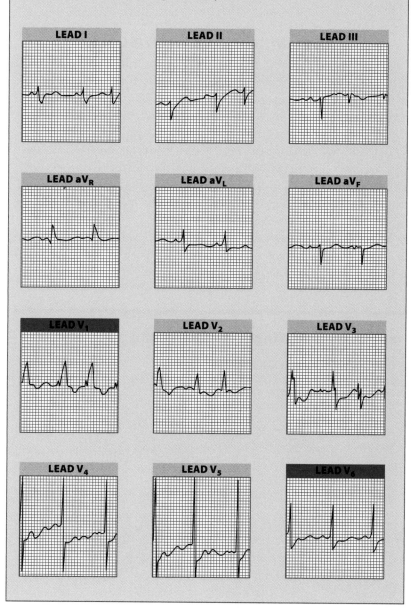

RBBB
(continued)

Lead V$_6$
+ Small Q wave then depolarization of left ventricle, producing tall R wave
+ Depolarization of right ventricle causes broad S wave
+ T wave positive

LBBB
+ Caused by hypertensive heart disease, aortic stenosis, degenerative changes of conduction system, or CAD
+ QRS complex > 0.12 second

Lead V$_1$
+ Depolarization spreads from right ventricle to left, producing S wave with positive T wave
+ S wave may follow Q wave or small R wave

Lead V$_6$
+ No initial Q wave occurs
+ Tall, notched R wave appears as impulse spreads from right to left with negative T wave

the negative deflection is called a secondary T-wave change and isn't clinically significant.

The opposite occurs in lead V$_6$. A small Q wave is followed by depolarization of the left ventricle, which produces a tall R wave. Depolarization of the right ventricle then causes a broad S wave. In lead V$_6$, the T wave should be positive.

LEFT BUNDLE-BRANCH BLOCK

Left bundle-branch block (LBBB) never occurs normally. This block is usually caused by hypertensive heart disease, aortic stenosis, degenerative changes of the conduction system, or CAD. (See *Understanding LBBB*.) When it occurs along with an anterior wall MI, if complete heart block occurs, it may require insertion of a pacemaker.

In LBBB, the QRS complex will be greater than 0.12 second because the ventricles are activated sequentially, not simultaneously. (See *Recognizing LBBB*.) As the wave of depolarization spreads from the right ventricle to the left, a wide S wave is produced in lead V$_1$, with a positive T wave. The S wave may be preceded by a Q wave or a small R wave.

In lead V$_6$, no initial Q wave occurs. A tall, notched R wave, or a slurred one, is produced as the impulse spreads from right to left. This initial positive deflection is a sign of LBBB. The T wave is negative.

Understanding LBBB

In left bundle-branch block (LBBB), the impulse first travels down the right bundle branch (arrow 1). Then the impulse activates the interventricular septum from right to left (arrow 2), the opposite of normal activation. Finally, the impulse activates the left ventricle (arrow 3).

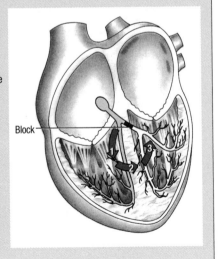

Recognizing LBBB

This 12-lead ECG shows characteristic changes of a left bundle-branch block (LBBB). All leads have prolonged QRS complexes. In lead V_1, note the QS wave pattern. In lead V_6, you'll see the slurred R wave and T-wave inversion. The elevated ST segments and upright T waves in leads V_1 to V_4 are also common in LBBB.

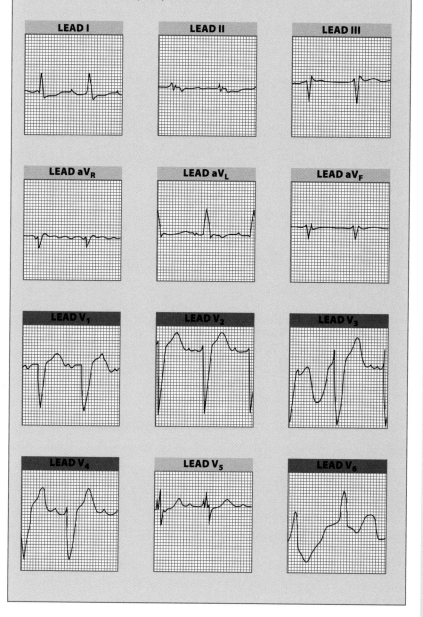

Distinguishing BBB from WPW syndrome

Wolff-Parkinson-White (WPW) syndrome is a common type of preexcitation syndrome, an abnormal condition in which electrical impulses enter the ventricles from the atria by using an accessory pathway that bypasses the atrioventricular (AV) junction. This results in a short PR interval and a wide QRS complex with an initial slurring of the upward slope of the QRS complex, called a delta wave. Because the delta wave prolongs the QRS complex, its presence may be confused with a bundle-branch block (BBB).

BUNDLE-BRANCH BLOCK
✦ Carefully examine the QRS complex, noting which part of the complex is widened. A BBB involves a defective conduction of electrical impulses through the right or left bundle branch from the bundle of His to the Purkinje network causing a right or left BBB.
✦ This conduction disturbance results in an overall increase in QRS duration, or widening of the last part of the QRS complex, while the initial part of the QRS complex commonly appears normal.
✦ Carefully examine the 12-lead ECG. With BBB, the prolonged duration of the QRS complexes will generally be consistent in all leads.
✦ Measure the PR interval. BBB has no effect on the PR interval, so the PR intervals are generally normal. Keep in mind, though, that if the patient has a preexisting AV conduction defect, such as first-degree AV block, the PR interval will be prolonged.

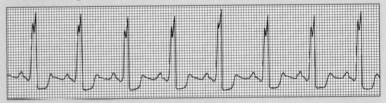

WOLFF-PARKINSON-WHITE SYNDROME
✦ A delta wave occurs at the beginning of the QRS complex, usually causing a distinctive slurring or hump in its initial slope. A delta wave isn't present in BBB.
✦ On the 12-lead ECG, the delta wave will be most pronounced in the leads "looking at" the part of the heart where the accessory pathway is located.
✦ The delta wave shortens the PR interval in WPW syndrome.

Short PR interval   Delta wave

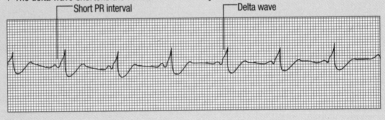

It may be difficult to tell the difference between BBB and Wolff-Parkinson-White (WPW) syndrome. (See *Distinguishing BBB from WPW syndrome.*) Whenever you spot BBB, check for WPW syndrome.

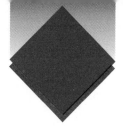

Appendices
Selected references
Index

Quick guide to arrhythmias

SINUS ARRHYTHMIA

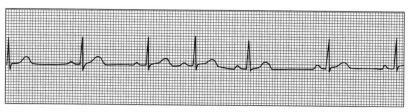

Features
+ Rhythm irregular; varies with respiratory cycle
+ Normal P wave preceding each QRS complex
+ P-P and R-R intervals shorter during inspiration and longer during expiration

Causes
+ Normal variation in athletes, children, and older adults
+ Digoxin or morphine use, increased intracranial pressure (ICP), and inferior wall myocardial infarction (MI)

Treatment
+ Typically no treatment necessary; possible correction of underlying cause

SINUS TACHYCARDIA

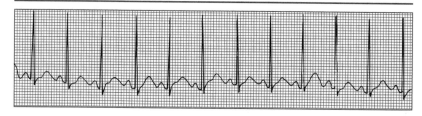

Features
+ Rhythm regular
+ Atrial and ventricular rates equal; rate > 100 beats/minute
+ Normal P wave preceding each normal QRS complex

Causes
+ Normal physiologic response to fever, exercise, stress, fear, anxiety, pain, dehydration; may accompany shock, left-sided heart failure, pericarditis, hyperthyroidism, anemia, pulmonary embolism, or sepsis

◆ Atropine, isoproterenol, aminophylline, dopamine, dobutamine, epinephrine, quinidine, caffeine, alcohol, amphetamine, or nicotine use

Treatment
◆ No treatment necessary if patient is asymptomatic
◆ Correction of underlying cause
◆ Beta-adrenergic or calcium channel blocker administration, if cardiac ischemia occurs

---

SINUS BRADYCARDIA

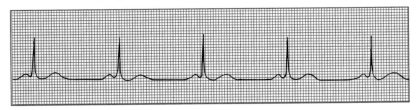

Features
◆ Rhythm regular
◆ Rate < 60 beats/minute
◆ Normal P wave preceding each normal QRS complex

Causes
◆ Normal during sleep and in well-conditioned heart (such as in athletes)
◆ Increased ICP, Valsalva's maneuver, carotid sinus massage, vomiting, hypothyroidism, hyperkalemia, hypothermia, cardiomyopathy, or inferior wall MI
◆ Beta-adrenergic blocker, calcium channel blocker, lithium, sotalol, amiodarone, digoxin, or quinidine use

Treatment
◆ No treatment needed (patient is usually asymptomatic); if drugs are cause, possibly discontinuation of use
◆ Atropine administration for low cardiac output, dizziness, weakness, altered level of consciousness, or low blood pressure
◆ Dopamine or epinephrine infusion, if indicated
◆ Temporary or permanent pacemaker may be needed

SINUS ARREST

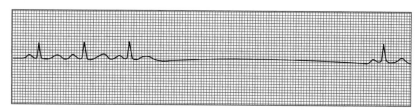

Features

+ Rhythm regular, except for missing PQRST complexes (irregular as result of missing complexes)
+ PQRST complex missing during arrest, when present normal P wave precedes each normal QRS complex.

Causes

+ Coronary artery disease (CAD), acute myocarditis, or acute inferior wall MI
+ Increased vagal tone (Valsalva's maneuver, carotid sinus massage, or vomiting)
+ Digoxin, quinidine, procainamide, or salicylate use (especially if given at toxic levels)
+ Excessive doses of beta-adrenergic blockers
+ Sinus node disease

Treatment

+ No treatment needed, if patient is asymptomatic
+ For mild symptoms, possible discontinuation of drugs that contribute to arrhythmia
+ Atropine administration, if patient is symptomatic
+ Temporary or permanent pacemaker for repeated episodes

PREMATURE ATRIAL CONTRACTIONS (PACs)

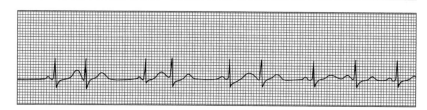

Features

+ Premature, abnormal P waves (differ in configuration from normal P waves)
+ QRS complexes after P waves, except in blocked PACs
+ P wave often buried or identified in preceding T wave

Causes

+ Triggered by alcohol or cigarette use, anxiety, fever, or infectious disease in normal heart

+ Heart failure, coronary or valvular heart disease, acute respiratory failure, chronic obstructive pulmonary disease (COPD), electrolyte imbalance, or hypoxia
+ Digoxin toxicity

Treatment
+ No treatment needed, if patient is asymptomatic
+ Beta-adrenergic blockers or calcium channel blockers, if occurs frequently
+ Treatment of underlying cause; avoidance of triggers (caffeine or smoking) and use of stress-reduction measures

ATRIAL TACHYCARDIA

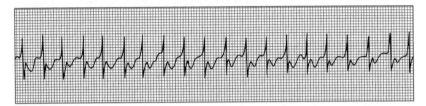

Features
+ Rhythm regular if block is constant; irregular if not
+ Rate 150 to 250 beats/minute
+ P waves regular but hidden in preceding T wave; precede QRS complexes

Causes
+ Physical or psychological stress, hypoxia, electrolyte imbalances, cardiomyopathy, congenital anomalies, MI, valvular disease, Wolff-Parkinson-White syndrome, cor pulmonale, hyperthyroidism, or systemic hypertension
+ Digoxin toxicity; caffeine, marijuana, or stimulant use

Treatment
+ Vagal stimulation and adenosine
+ Calcium channel blocker, beta-adrenergic blocker, amiodarone, procainamide, sotalol,or digoxin administration
+ Atrial overdrive pacing
+ If other treatments fail, synchronized cardioversion may be considered

ATRIAL FLUTTER

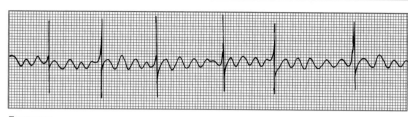

Features

+ Atrial rhythm regular; ventricular rhythm variable, depending on degree of atrioventricular (AV) block
+ Atrial rate 250 to 400 beats/minute; ventricular rate depends on degree of AV block
+ Sawtooth P-wave configuration (known as flutter or F waves)
+ QRS complexes uniform in shape

Causes

+ Heart failure, severe mitral valve disease, hyperthyroidism, pericardial disease, COPD, systemic arterial hypoxia, and acute MI

Treatment

+ Calcium channel blocker or beta-adrenergic blocker administration, if stable and heart functions normally
+ Amiodarone, ibutilide, flecainide, propafenone, or procainamide administration, if arrhythmia is present for less than 48 hours
+ Synchronized cardioversion immediately if patient is unstable
+ Anticoagulation prior to cardioversion, if arrhythmia is present for more than 48 hours
+ Ablation therapy for recurrent rhythm

ATRIAL FIBRILLATION

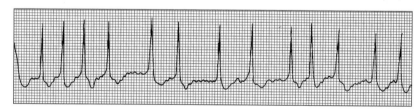

Features

+ Atrial and ventricular rhythm grossly irregular
+ Atrial rate > than 400 beats/minute; ventricular rate varies
+ No P waves; replaced by fine fibrillatory waves
+ No PR interval
+ QRS complexes uniform in configuration and duration

Causes
+ Ischemic heart disease, hypertension, heart failure, valvular heart disease, and rheumatic heart disease
+ Diabetes
+ Alcohol abuse
+ Thyroid disorders
+ Lung and pleural disorders

Treatment
+ Follow treatment guidelines for atrial flutter

JUNCTIONAL ESCAPE RHYTHM

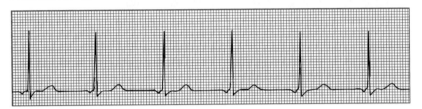

Features
+ Rhythm regular
+ Rate 40 to 60 beats/minute
+ P waves before, hidden in, or after QRS complex; inverted if visible
+ PR interval < 0.12 second (measurable only if P wave appears before QRS complex)
+ QRS configuration and duration normal

Causes
+ Inferior wall MI and rheumatic heart
+ Digoxin toxicity
+ Sick sinus syndrome
+ Vagal stimulation

Treatment
+ Treatment of underlying cause
+ Atropine administration, for symptomatic slow rate
+ Pacemaker insertion, if refractory to drugs
+ Discontinuation of digoxin, if appropriate

PREMATURE JUNCTIONAL CONTRACTIONS

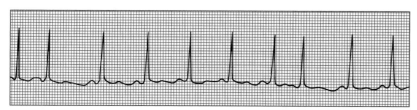

Features
+ Rhythm irregular
+ P waves before, hidden in, or after QRS complexes; inverted if visible
+ PR interval < 0.12 second, if P wave precedes QRS complex
+ QRS configuration and duration normal

Causes
+ Inferior wall MI or ischemia, swelling of AV junction after surgery, rheumatic heart disease, and valvular disease
+ Digoxin toxicity (most common) and excessive caffeine intake

Treatment
+ No treatment if patient is asymptomatic
+ Correction of underlying cause
+ Discontinuation of digoxin, if appropriate
+ Possible elimination of caffeine

JUNCTIONAL TACHYCARDIA

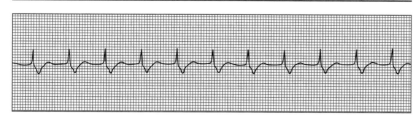

Features
+ Rhythm regular
+ Rate 100 to 200 beats/minute
+ P wave before, hidden in, or after QRS complex; inverted if visible
+ QRS configuration and duration normal

Causes
+ Congenital heart disease (in children)
+ Digoxin toxicity
+ Swelling of AV junction after heart surgery
+ Inferior- or posterior-wall MI or ischemia

Treatment

◆ Correction of underlying cause

◆ Discontinuation of digoxin, if appropriate

◆ Vagal maneuvers, adenosine, amiodarone, beta-adrenergic blocker, or calcium channel blocker, to slow rate

◆ Ablation therapy, if recurrent, followed by permanent pacemaker insertion

WANDERING PACEMAKER

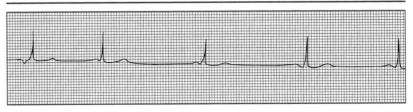

Features

◆ Rhythm irregular

◆ P waves change in configuration, indicating origin in sinoatrial node, atria, or AV junction (*Hallmark:* At least three different P wave configurations)

◆ PR interval varies

◆ QRS configuration and duration normal

Causes

◆ May be normal in young patients, common in athletes with slow heart rates

◆ Increased vagal tone

◆ Digoxin toxicity

◆ Inflammation of atrial tissue, valvular heart disease

Treatment

◆ No treatment, if patient is asymptomatic

◆ Treatment of underlying cause, if patient is symptomatic

FIRST-DEGREE AV BLOCK

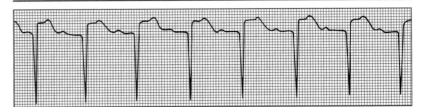

Features

◆ Rhythm regular

◆ P wave preceding each QRS complex; QRS complex normal

◆ PR interval > 0.20 second and constant

Causes

✦ May occur in healthy person

✦ Myocardial ischemia or infarction, myocarditis, or degenerative heart changes

✦ Digoxin, calcium channel blocker, and beta-adrenergic blocker use

Treatment

✦ Cautious use of digoxin, calcium channel blockers, and beta-adrenergic blockers

✦ Correction of underlying cause

SECOND-DEGREE AV BLOCK TYPE I (MOBITZ I, WENCKEBACH)

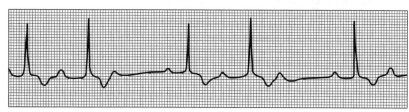

Features

✦ Atrial rhythm regular

✦ Ventricular rhythm irregular

✦ Atrial rate exceeds ventricular rate

✦ PR interval progressively, but only slightly, longer with each cycle until a P wave appears without a QRS complex

Causes

✦ Inferior wall MI, CAD, rheumatic fever, or vagal stimulation

✦ Digoxin toxicity

✦ Propranolol or verapamil use

Treatment

✦ Treatment of underlying cause

✦ Atropine administration or temporary pacemaker, for symptomatic bradycardia

✦ Discontinuation of digoxin, if appropriate

SECOND-DEGREE AV BLOCK TYPE II (MOBITZ TYPE II)

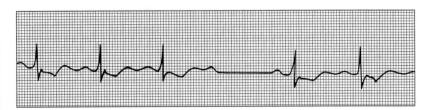

Features
+ Atrial rhythm regular
+ Ventricular rhythm possibly irregular, varying with degree of block
+ P waves normal size, some not followed by a QRS complex
+ PR interval is constant for conducted beats
+ QRS complexes periodically absent

Causes
+ Severe CAD, anterior MI, or degenerative changes in conduction system
+ Digoxin toxicity

Treatment
+ Treatment of underlying cause
+ Atropine, dopamine, or epinephrine administration, for symptomatic bradycardia (use atropine cautiously, it may worsen ischemia with MI)
+ Temporary or permanent pacemaker
+ Discontinuation of digoxin, if appropriate

THIRD-DEGREE AV BLOCK (COMPLETE HEART BLOCK)

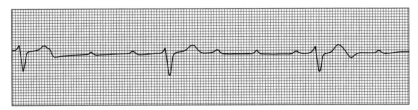

Features
+ Atrial rhythm regular
+ Ventricular rhythm regular and rate slow; if escape rhythm originates in AV node, rate is 40 to 60 beats/minute; if it originates in Purkinje system, rate is < 40 beats/minute
+ No relationship between P waves and QRS complexes
+ PR interval can't be measured
+ QRS complex normal (originating in AV node) or wide and bizarre (originating in Purkinje system)

Causes

+ Inferior or anterior wall MI, CAD, degenerative changes in heart, congenital abnormality, or hypoxia
+ Digoxin toxicity

Treatment

+ Treatment of underlying cause
+ Atropine, dopamine, or epinephrine administration, for symptomatic bradycardia (*Note:* Don't use atropine with wide QRS complexes.)
+ Temporary (transcutaneous or transvenous) or permanent pacemaker

PREMATURE VENTRICULAR CONTRACTIONS (PVCs)

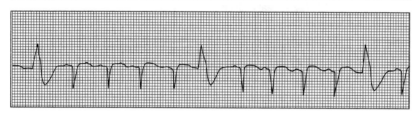

Features

+ Atrial and ventricular rhythms may be regular in underlying rhythm; irregular during PVCs
+ QRS premature
+ QRS complex wide and bizarre, usually > than 0.12 second in premature beat
+ T wave opposite direction to QRS complex
+ PVCs may occur singly, in pairs, or in threes; alternating with normal beats; possibly unifocal or multifocal
+ Most ominous when clustered, multifocal, and with R wave on T pattern
+ PVC may be followed by full or incomplete compensatory pause

Causes

+ Heart failure; myocardial ischemia, infarction, or contusion; myocarditis, myocardial irritation by ventricular catheter (such as pacemaker); hypokalemia; hypomagnesemia; metabolic acidosis; or hypocalcemia
+ Drug intoxication, particularly with cocaine, tricyclic antidepressants, and amphetamines
+ Caffeine, tobacco, or alcohol use
+ Psychological stress, anxiety, pain, or exercise

Treatment

+ If warranted, amiodarone, procainamide, or lidocaine administration
+ Treatment of underlying cause
+ Discontinuation of drug causing toxicity
+ Potassium chloride I.V., if induced by hypokalemia
+ Magnesium replacement, if due to hypomagnesemia

VENTRICULAR TACHYCARDIA

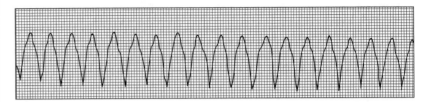

Features
+ Atrial rhythm can't be determined; ventricular rhythm usually regular, may be slightly irregular
+ Ventricular rate 100 to 250 beats/minute
+ P waves indiscernible
+ QRS complexes wide and bizarre; duration > 0.12 second
+ May start and stop suddenly

Causes
+ Myocardial ischemia, or infarction, CAD; valvular heart disease; heart failure; cardiomyopathy; ventricular catheterization; hypokalemia; hypercalcemia; or pulmonary embolism
+ Digoxin, procainamide, quinidine, or cocaine toxicity

Treatment
+ For monomorphic ventricular tachycardia: procainamide, sotalol, amiodarone, or lidocaine administration, using Advanced Cardiac Life Support (ACLS) protocol; if unsuccessful, cardioversion
+ For polymorphic ventricular tachycardia with normal QT interval: beta-adrenergic blocker, lidocaine, amiodarone, procainamide, or sotalol administration, using ACLS protocol; if unsuccessful, cardioversion
+ For polymorphic ventricular tachycardia with prolonged QT interval: magnesium I.V. administration, overdrive pacing if rhythm persists; possibly phenytoin, isoproterenol, or lidocaine administration
+ For pulselessness: initiation of cardiopulmonary resuscitation (CPR) followed by treatment for ventricular fibrillation
+ Implantable cardioverter-defibrillator, if recurrent ventricular tachycardia

VENTRICULAR FIBRILLATION

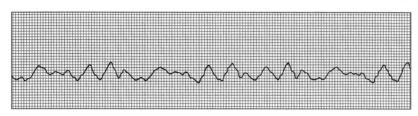

Features
+ Ventricular rhythm rapid and chaotic
+ No discernible P waves, QRS complexes, or T waves
+ Fine or coarse fibrillatory waves

Causes
+ Myocardial ischemia or infarction, untreated ventricular tachycardia, hypokalemia, acid-base imbalances, hyperkalemia, hypercalcemia, electric shock, or severe hypothermia
+ Digoxin, epinephrine, or quinidine toxicity

Treatment
+ CPR; ACLS protocol for defibrillation
+ Endotracheal intubation
+ Epinephrine or vasopressin administration, or amiodarone or lidocaine administration, if ineffective, magnesium sulfate or procainamide administration
+ Implantable cardioverter-defibrillator, if at risk for recurrent ventricular fibrillation

ASYSTOLE

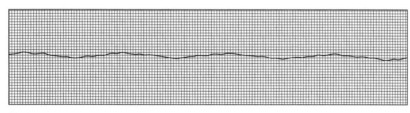

Features
+ No atrial or ventricular rate or rhythm
+ No discernible P waves, QRS complexes, or T waves

Causes
+ Myocardial ischemia or infarction, heart failure, prolonged hypoxemia, severe electrolyte disturbances (such as hyperkalemia), severe acid-base disturbances, electric shock, ventricular arrhythmias, AV block, pulmonary embolism, or cardiac tamponade
+ Cocaine overdose

Treatment
+ After verification of rhythm (by checking more than one lead), CPR (following ACLS protocol)
+ Endotracheal intubation
+ Transcutaneous pacemaker
+ Treatment of underlying cause
+ Repeated doses of epinephrine and atropine, as ordered

Guide to cardiovascular drugs

This chart details the drugs most commonly used to improve cardiovascular function, including indications, and special considerations for each.

DRUGS	INDICATIONS	SPECIAL CONSIDERATIONS
ADRENERGIC BLOCKERS		
Alpha-adrenergic blockers Phentolamine, prazosin	✦ Hypertension ✦ Peripheral vascular disorders ✦ Pheochromocytoma	✦ Monitor vital signs and heart rhythm before, during, and after administration. ✦ Instruct the patient to rise slowly to a standing position to avoid orthostatic hypotension. ✦ Assess pulse rate before administering dose.
Beta-adrenergic blockers *Nonselective* Carvedilol, labetalol, nadolol, penbutolol, pindolol, propranolol, sotalol, timolol *Selective* Acebutolol, atenolol, betaxolol, bisoprolol, esmolol, metoprolol	✦ Prevention of complications after myocardial infarction (MI), angina, hypertension, supraventricular arrhythmias (such as paroxysmal supraventricular tachycardia), anxiety, essential tremor, cardiovascular symptoms associated with thyrotoxicosis, migraine headaches, pheochromocytoma	✦ Monitor apical pulse rate before administration. Monitor blood pressure, electrocardiogram (ECG), and heart rate and rhythm frequently. ✦ Beta-adrenergic blockers can alter the requirements for insulin and oral antidiabetic agents. ✦ Signs of hypoglycemic shock may be masked; watch patients with diabetes for sweating, fatigue, and hunger.
ADRENERGICS		
Catecholamines Dobutamine	✦ Increase cardiac output in short-term treatment of cardiac decompensation from depressed contractility	✦ Monitor cardiac rate and rhythm and blood pressure carefully when initiating therapy or increasing the dose. ✦ Correct hypovolemia before administering drug. ✦ Incompatible with alkaline solution (sodium bicarbonate); don't mix or give through same line, and don't mix with other drugs. ✦ Administer continuous drip on infusion pump. ✦ Give drug into a large vein to prevent irritation or extravasation at site.

DRUGS	INDICATIONS	SPECIAL CONSIDERATIONS
ADRENERGICS *(continued)*		
Catecholamines (continued) Dopamine	✦ Adjunct in shock to increase cardiac output, blood pressure, and urine flow	✦ Monitor cardiac rate and rhythm and blood pressure carefully when initiating therapy or increasing the dose. ✦ Correct hypovolemia before administering drug. ✦ Incompatible with alkaline solution (sodium bicarbonate); don't mix or give through same line, and don't mix with other drugs. ✦ Administer continuous drip on infusion pump. ✦ Give drug into a large vein to prevent extravasation; if extravasation occurs, stop infusion and treat site with phentolamine infiltrate to prevent tissue necrosis.
Epinephrine	✦ Bronchospasm ✦ Hypersensitivity reactions ✦ Anaphylaxis ✦ Restoration of cardiac rhythm in cardiac arrest	✦ Monitor cardiac rate and rhythm and blood pressure carefully when initiating therapy or increasing the dose. ✦ Correct hypovolemia before administering drug. ✦ Incompatible with alkaline solution (sodium bicarbonate); don't mix or give through same line, and don't mix with other drugs. ✦ Administer continuous drip on infusion pump. ✦ Give drug into a large vein to prevent irritation or extravasation at site.
Norepinephrine	✦ Maintain blood pressure in acute hypotensive states ✦ GI bleeding	✦ Monitor cardiac rate and rhythm and blood pressure carefully when initiating therapy or increasing the dose. ✦ Correct hypovolemia before administering drug. ✦ Incompatible with alkaline solution (sodium bicarbonate); don't mix or give through same line, and don't mix with other drugs. ✦ Administer continuous drip on infusion pump; can be given by I.V. push in cardiac arrest situations. ✦ Give drug into a large vein to prevent extravasation; if extravasation occurs, stop infusion and treat site with phentolamine infiltrate to prevent tissue necrosis.
Noncatecholamines Ephedrine	✦ Maintain blood pressure in acute hypotensive states, especially with spinal anesthesia ✦ Treatment of orthostatic hypotension and bronchospasm	✦ Monitor cardiac rate and rhythm and blood pressure carefully when initiating therapy or increasing the dose. ✦ Correct hypovolemia before administering drug. ✦ Give drug into a large vein to prevent irritation or extravasation at site.

DRUGS	INDICATIONS	SPECIAL CONSIDERATIONS
Noncatecholamines *(continued)*		
Phenylephrine	✦ Maintain blood pressure in hypotensive states, especially hypotensive emergencies with spinal anesthesia	✦ Monitor cardiac rate and rhythm and blood pressure carefully when initiating therapy or increasing the dose. ✦ Correct hypovolemia before administering drug. ✦ Don't mix with other drugs. ✦ Administer continuous drip on infusion pump. ✦ Give drug into a large vein to prevent extravasation; if extravasation occurs, stop infusion and treat site with phentolamine infiltrate to prevent tissue necrosis.

ANTIANGINAL DRUGS

DRUGS	INDICATIONS	SPECIAL CONSIDERATIONS
Nitrates Isosorbide dinitrate, isosorbide mononitrate, nitroglycerin	✦ Relief and prevention of angina	✦ Monitor the patient's blood pressure before and after administration. ✦ Only sublingual and translingual forms should be used.
Calcium channel blockers Amlodipine, diltiazem, nicardipine, nifedipine, verapamil	✦ Long-term prevention of angina (especially Prinzmetal's angina)	✦ Monitor cardiac rate and rhythm and blood pressure carefully when initiating therapy or increasing the dose. ✦ Calcium supplementation may decrease the effects of calcium channel blockers.

ANTIARRHYTHMICS

DRUGS	INDICATIONS	SPECIAL CONSIDERATIONS
Class IA antiarrhythmics Disopyramide phosphate, procainamide hydrochloride, quinidine sulfate, quinidine gluconate	✦ Ventricular tachycardia ✦ Atrial fibrillation ✦ Atrial flutter ✦ Paroxysmal atrial tachycardia (PAT)	✦ Check apical pulse rate before therapy. If you note extremes in pulse rate, withhold the dose and notify the physician. ✦ Use cautiously in patients with asthma. ✦ Monitor for ECG changes (widening QRS complexes, prolonged QT interval).
Class IB antiarrhythmics Lidocaine, mexiletine, tocainide	✦ Ventricular tachycardia ✦ Ventricular fibrillation	✦ IB antiarrhythmics may potentiate the effects of others. ✦ Administer I.V. infusions using an infusion pump. ✦ Monitor for ECG changes (widening QRS complexes, prolonged PR interval).
Class IC antiarrhythmics Flecainide, moricizine, propafenone	✦ Ventricular tachycardia ✦ Ventricular fibrillation ✦ Supraventricular arrhythmias	✦ Correct electrolyte imbalances before administration. ✦ Monitor the patient's ECG before and after dosage adjustments. ✦ Monitor for ECG changes (widening QRS complexes, prolonged PR and QT interval).

DRUGS	INDICATIONS	SPECIAL CONSIDERATIONS
ANTIARRHYTHMICS (continued)		
Class II antiarrhythmics Acebutolol, esmolol, propranolol	✦ Atrial flutter ✦ Atrial fibrillation ✦ PAT	✦ Monitor apical heart rate and blood pressure. ✦ Abruptly stopping these drugs can exacerbate angina and precipitate MI. ✦ Monitor for ECG changes (prolonged PR interval).
Class III antiarrhythmics Amiodarone, dofetilide, ibutilide, sotalol	✦ Life-threatening arrhythmias resistant to other antiarrhythmics	✦ Amiodarone increases the risk of digoxin toxicity in patients also taking digoxin. ✦ Monitor for signs of pulmonary toxicity (dyspnea, nonproductive cough, and pleuritic chest pain) in patients taking amiodarone. ✦ Monitor blood pressure, heart rate, and rhythm for changes. ✦ Monitor ECG before and after dosage adjustments. ✦ Monitor for ECG changes (prolonged QT interval) in patients taking dofetilide, ibutilide, and sotalol.
Class IV antiarrhythmics Diltiazem, verapamil	✦ Supraventricular arrhythmias	✦ Monitor heart rate and rhythm and blood pressure carefully when initiating therapy or increasing dose. ✦ Calcium supplements may reduce effectiveness.
Miscellaneous Adenosine	✦ Paroxysmal supraventricular tachycardia	✦ Adenosine must be administered over 1 to 2 seconds, followed by a 20-ml flush of normal saline solution. ✦ Record rhythm strip during administration. ✦ A brief period of asystole (up to 15 seconds) may occur after rapid administration.
ANTICOAGULANTS		
Heparins Heparin and low-molecular-weight heparins, such as dalteparin and enoxaparin	✦ Deep vein thrombosis ✦ Embolism prophylaxis ✦ Disseminated intravascular coagulation ✦ Prevention of complications after MI	✦ Monitor partial thromboplastin time (PTT); the therapeutic range is 1½ to 2½ times the control. ✦ Monitor the patient for signs of bleeding. ✦ Concomitant administration with nonsteroidal anti-inflammatory drugs, iron dextran, or an antiplatelet drug increases the risk of bleeding. ✦ Protamine sulfate reverses the effects of heparin.

DRUGS	INDICATIONS	SPECIAL CONSIDERATIONS
ANTICOAGULANTS *(continued)*		
Oral anticoagulants Warfarin	✦ Deep vein thrombosis prophylaxis ✦ Prevention of complications of prosthetic heart valves or diseased mitral valves ✦ Atrial arrhythmias, such as atrial fibrillation and atrial flutter	✦ Monitor prothrombin time (PT) and International Normalized Ratio (INR) in patients receiving warfarin; the effects of oral anticoagulants can be reversed with phytonadione (vitamin K_1). ✦ Monitor the patient for signs of bleeding.
Antiplatelet drugs Aspirin, dipyridamole, sulfinpyrazone, ticlopidine	✦ Decreased risk of death post-MI ✦ Prevention of complications of prosthetic heart valves	✦ Monitor the patient for signs of bleeding. ✦ Aspirin, sulfinpyrazone, and ticlopidine should be taken with meals to prevent GI irritation. ✦ Dipyridamole should be taken with a full glass of fluid at least 1 hour before meals.
ANTIHYPERTENSIVES		
Vasodilators Diazoxide, hydralazine, minoxidil, nitroprusside	✦ Moderate to severe hypertension (in combination with other drugs)	✦ Monitor blood pressure before and after administration.
Angiotensin-converting enzyme inhibitors Benazepril, captopril, enalapril, enalaprilat, fosinopril, lisinopril, moexipril, perindopril, quinapril, ramipril,trandolapril	✦ Hypertension ✦ Heart failure	✦ Monitor blood pressure before and after administration. ✦ In patients whose renal function may depend on the renin-angiotensin-aldosterone system, such as those with severe heart failure, treatment with angiotensin-converting enzyme (ACE) inhibitors and angiotensin-receptor blockers has been related to oliguria or progressive azotemia and (rarely) to acute renal failure or death.
Angiotensin II receptor blockers Candesartan, eprosartan, irbesartan, losartan, olmesartan, telmisartan, valsartan	✦ Hypertension ✦ Valvular disease	✦ Monitor blood pressure before and after administration. ✦ In patients whose renal function may depend on the renin-angiotensin-aldosterone system, such as those with severe heart failure, treatment with ACE inhibitors and angiotensin-receptor blockers has been related to oliguria or progressive azotemia and (rarely) to acute renal failure or death.

DRUGS	INDICATIONS	SPECIAL CONSIDERATIONS
ANTILIPEMICS		
Bile-sequestering drugs Cholestyramine, coleseve- lam, colestipol	✦ Hyperlipidemia ✦ Hypercholesterolemia	✦ Monitor blood cholesterol and lipid levels before and peri- odically during therapy. ✦ Monitor liver function studies and creatine kinase (CK) throughout therapy. ✦ Advise the patient to drink 2 to 3 qt (2 to 3 L) of fluid daily and to report persistent or severe constipation.
Fibric acid dirivatives Fenofibrate, gemfibrozil	✦ Hyperlipidemia ✦ Hypercholesterolemia ✦ Hypertryglyceridemia	✦ Monitor blood cholesterol and lipid levels before and peri- odically during therapy. ✦ Monitor liver function studies and CK throughout therapy. ✦ Advise the patient to drink 2 to 3 qt (2 to 3 L) of fluid daily and to report persistent or severe constipation.
HMG CoA inhibitors Atorvastatin, fluvastatin, lovastatin, pravastatin, sim- vastatin	✦ Hyperlipidemia (types IV and V)	• If being administered with bile sequestrants, give at least 4 to 6 hours apart. • Administer with meals (or at bedtime when using ex- tended release forms). ✦ Monitor blood cholesterol and lipid levels before and peri- odically during therapy. ✦Monitor liver function and CK levels throughout therapy.
CARDIAC GLYCOSIDE AND PHOSPHODIESTERASE (PDE) INHIBITORS		
Cardiac glycoside Digoxin	✦ Heart failure ✦ Supraventricular arrhythmias	✦ If immediate effects are required, a loading dose of digoxin is required. ✦ Check apical pulse for 1 minute before administration; report pulse less than 60 beats/minute. ✦ Therapeutic serum levels are 0.5 to 2 ng/ml.
PDE inhibitors Inamrinone, milrinone	✦ Heart failure refractory to digoxin, diuretics, and vasodilators	✦ These drugs are contraindicated in the acute phase of MI and after MI. ✦ Serum potassium levels should be within normal limits before and during therapy.

DRUGS	INDICATIONS	SPECIAL CONSIDERATIONS
DIURETICS		
Thiazide and thiazide-like diuretics Bendroflumethiazide, chlorthalidone, chlorothiazide, hydrochlorothiazide, hydroflumethiazide, indapamide	✦ Hypertension ✦ Edema	✦ Monitor serum potassium levels. ✦ Monitor intake and output. ✦ Monitor blood glucose values in patients with diabetes. Thiazide diuretics can cause hyperglycemia.
Loop diuretics Bumetanide, ethacrynic acid, furosemide	✦ Hypertension ✦ Heart failure ✦ Edema	✦ Monitor for signs of excess diuresis (hypotension, tachycardia, poor skin turgor, and excessive thirst). ✦ Monitor blood pressure, heart rate, and intake and output. ✦ Monitor serum electrolyte levels.
Potassium-sparing diuretics Amiloride, spironolactone, triamterene	✦ Edema ✦ Diuretic-induced hypokalemia in patients with heart failure ✦ Hypertension	✦ Monitor ECG for arrhythmias. ✦ Monitor serum potassium levels. ✦ Monitor intake and output.
THROMBOLYTICS		
Alteplase, reteplase, streptokinase	✦ Acute MI ✦ Acute ischemic stroke ✦ Pulmonary embolus ✦ Catheter occlusion ✦ Arterial thrombosis	✦ Monitor PTT, PT, INR, hemoglobin, and hematocrit before, during, and after administration. ✦ Monitor vital signs frequently during and immediately after administration. Don't use an automatic blood pressure cuff to monitor blood pressure. ✦ Monitor puncture sites for bleeding. ✦ Monitor for signs of bleeding. ✦ Monitor for reperfusion arrhythmias when used to treat acute MI.

Selected references

Aehlert, B. *ACLS Quick Review Study Guide,* 2nd ed. St. Louis: Mosby–Year Book, Inc., 2002.

Albert, N.M. "Cardiac Resynchronization Therapy through Biventricular Pacing in Patients with Heart Failure and Ventricular Dyssynchrony," *Critical Care Nurse* 23(3 Suppl.):2-13, June 2003.

American Heart Association. "Guidelines 2000 for Cardiopulmonary Resuscitation and Emergency Cardiovascular Care," *Circulation* 102(suppl 8): 11-165, August 2000.

Catalano, J. *Guide to ECG Analysis,* 2nd ed. Philadelphia: Lippincott Williams & Wilkins, 2002.

Conover, M.B. *Understanding Electrocardiography,* 8th ed. St. Louis: Mosby–Year Book, Inc., 2002.

Cosio, F.G., and Delpon, E. "New Antiarrhythmic Drugs for Atrial Flutter and Atrial Fibrillation: A Conceptual Breakthrough at Last?" *Circulation* 105(3):276-78, January 2002.

Cummins, R.O. (Ed). *ACLS: Principles and Practice.* Dallas: American Heart Association, 2003.

ECG Cards, 4th ed. Philadelphia: Lippincott Williams & Wilkins, 2005.

ECG Interpretation Made Incredibly Easy, 3rd ed. Philadelphia: Lippincott Williams & Wilkins, 2005.

Mastering ACLS, 2nd ed. Philadelphia: Lippincott Williams & Wilkins, 2005.

McAlister, F.A. "Atrial fibrillation, Shared Decision Making, and the Prevention of Stroke," *Stroke* 33(1):243-44, January 2002.

Wagner, G.S. *Marriott's Practical Electrocardiography,* 10th ed. Philadelphia: Lippincott Williams & Wilkins, 2001.

Woods, S., et al. *Cardiac Nursing,* 5th ed. Philadelphia: Lippincott Williams & Wilkins, 2005.

Index

i refers to an illustration; t refers to a table; **boldface** indicates color pages.

i refers to an illustration; t refers to a table; **boldface** indicates color pages.

i refers to an illustration; t refers to a table; **boldface** indicates color pages.

i refers to an illustration; t refers to a table; **boldface** indicates color pages.

i refers to an illustration; t refers to a table; **boldface** indicates color pages.

i refers to an illustration; t refers to a table; **boldface** indicates color pages.

i refers to an illustration; t refers to a table; **boldface** indicates color pages.

i refers to an illustration; t refers to a table; **boldface** indicates color pages.

i refers to an illustration; t refers to a table; **boldface** indicates color pages.

i refers to an illustration; t refers to a table; **boldface** indicates color pages.

i refers to an illustration; t refers to a table; **boldface** indicates color pages.

---

i refers to an illustration; t refers to a table; **boldface** indicates color pages.